"Understanding how nutritional chemistry affects the mind has changed my life. Many patients have told me it changed theirs too. I think it is no exaggeration to claim this book contains information which can change your life for the better."

Dr. Lesser has found incontrovertible proof that you are what you eat . . . and where you live . . . and the water you drink.

Find out how foods you eat every day can cause serious allergic reactions that manifest in physical and emotional disturbances . . .

How aluminum cookware affects the nutritional value of your food . . .

Which mineral increases sexual staying power . . .

Which B vitamin promotes dreaming . . .

The facts about vitamin C . . .

Nutrition and Vitamin Therapy is the first book of its kind to take the mystery out of preventive medicine and nutrition and make the important facts accessible to everyone.

You need to know.

NUTRITION
AND
VITAMIN THERAPY

Michael Lesser, M.D.

BANTAM BOOKS
TORONTO · NEW YORK · LONDON · SYDNEY

*This low-priced Bantam Book
has been completely reset in a type face
designed for easy reading, and was printed
from new plates. It contains the complete
text of the original hard-cover edition.*
NOT ONE WORD HAS BEEN OMITTED.

🙢

NUTRITION AND VITAMIN THERAPY
*A Bantam Book / published by arrangement with
Grove Press, Inc.*

PRINTING HISTORY
*Grove Press edition published April 1980
3 printings through February 1981*

Excerpted in Your Good Health *under the title "Sex &
Nutrition"*
Bantam edition / June 1981

*Bantam Books are published by Bantam Books, Inc. Its trade-
mark, consisting of the words "Bantam Books" and the por-
trayal of a bantam, is Registered in U.S. Patent and Trademark
Office and in other countries. Marca Registrada. Bantam
Books, Inc., 666 Fifth Avenue, New York, New York 10103.*

PRINTED IN THE UNITED STATES OF AMERICA

0 9 8 7 6 5 4 3 2

This book is for my family. For my father, Samuel, my first and best teacher of human nature. For my mother, Edith, who always believed in G-d. To my wife, Deborah, the treasure of my life; and our son Eli. If he is representative of his generation, there will be a beautiful tomorrow.

Acknowledgments

First I thank Drs. Abram Hoffer and Humphrey Osmond, originators of megavitamin therapy. My special gratitude to Drs. Carl C. Pfeiffer, David Hawkins, Jose A. Yaryura-Tobias, and Allen Cott, my first teachers.

I applaud my contemporaries: Drs. Richard Kunin, Harvey Ross, Elizabeth Rees, and Bernard Rimland in California, Carl Reich and Glenn Green in Canada, Jack Ward, Moke Williams, Michael Schacter, and Michael Janson in the East, Gary Vickar in St. Louis, and the deceased but remembered Walter Alvarez and Robert Meiers.

I have learned from the allergists: Drs. Thoren Randolph, Ben Feingold, Marshall Mandell, Phyllis Saifer, and Charles McGee.

Special appreciation also to Dr. Roger Williams, Dr. Linus Pauling, Richard Hicks, Harry and Theda Shifs, Elaine Jacobsen, Anne Segerman, Peggy Spanel, Rosalind La Roche, Elizabeth Gentala, Thelma Thompson, Dr. Lendon Smith, Eric Baig, John Stroh, Dr. Louis Langman, Dr. Fugan Neziroglu, Laurence Lesser, Helene Wilcox, Mollie Starr Schriftman, Dr. Emmanuel Cheraskin, and Alexander Schauss.

My gratitude to the political warriors for nutrition: Senator George McGovern and his aides, Alan Stone, Chris Hitt, and Marshall Matz; California Senate Speaker James Mills, and his aide Derek Casady.

Thanks to Mary Roddy, Nick and Marianne Bosco, Dr. Stephen Langer, and Cynthia Frantz and Claire Risley, who helped me with the manuscript.

Finally I thank my patients, who never gave up and

taught me so much. My deepest regards to my editor at Grove Press, Alan Rinzler.

I recall so many others, but brevity does not permit me to mention them; I am thankful and hope this book will prove worthy of their generosity and trust.

Contents

Foreword

In the almost twenty years that I have worked at the national and international levels on world food issues, nothing has intrigued me more than the pioneering research and clinical practice that has begun to link what we eat to our mental well-being. According to the National Institute of Mental Health, 6.4 million Americans are under some form of mental health care, an estimated 10 percent of all Americans are in need of such care. That translates into over 20 million people. If further initiatives are undertaken along nutritional lines, I think we might discover that a significant number of mental health problems can be cured or prevented through better diet.

However, of all the areas of promising nutrition research and knowledge, the relationship between nutrition and mental health and development is the least funded and the least understood. Thus, recognizing the relationship between nutrition and mental health is still very much a struggle. Established scientific thinking remains weighted against those few who are seeking to understand the complex links between the food we consume and how we think and behave. I believe that the publication of this book will not only help the individuals who read it, but will also contribute to a better understanding of the science and a better relationship between the scientists and practitioners who are all striving to improve the mental health of the American people.

—SENATOR GEORGE S. MCGOVERN,
Senate Sub-Committee on Nutrition

Introduction

When I started practicing psychiatry according to traditional methods, I realized it wasn't going to work for all my patients. I had been trained to do psychoanalytically oriented psychotherapy and to prescribe drugs. But psychotherapy is a lengthy and expensive process, practical for only a few. Drugs were sometimes effective in smothering symptoms but did not treat the cause of most problems.

Simultaneously, I became aware of the importance of sound nutrition and a fit body for mental health. Most of us know of the deleterious effects of alcohol and drugs on our bodies. Less obvious but equally real are the subtle effects caused by coffee, tobacco, pollutants such as lead and mercury, food additives, and food intolerances. I came to realize that every vitamin, every mineral, and every food has a distinct and specific effect on our bodies, and consequently our mental function.

In the past ten years, I've explored ever more deeply this relationship between nutrition and the mind. I am now convinced that what we eat makes a crucial difference in how we feel. This book, written over the past three years, documents that relationship in as much detail as is currently possible.

Nutrition and vitamin therapy will not cure everything. Often it's not the main problem. But whether or not we are aware of it, nutrition does affect us all. Incredible though it may seem, correct nutrition can mean the difference between depression and good cheer, between sanity and insanity, even between law-abiding self-control and criminal behavior.

A chemical understanding of the mind was what Sigmund Freud sought at the turn of the century, before abandoning his search as premature. Freud died in 1939; but I feel confident that were he alive today, he would be keenly interested in the developments of nutrition and vitamin therapy.

I do not wish to engage in conflict. Psychotherapy has its place, as does the judicious use of tranquilizers. What I do wish is to present a comprehensive picture of the benefits of nutrition and vitamin therapy. I am not saying we should all rush to the health food store and start gobbling megadoses of myriad vitamin capsules. But I do believe that nutrition and vitamin therapy presents the first and often the best treatment for much disease, of both the mind and body.

The cases presented in this book are true. If some of the stories seem too miraculous to be real, I say that "truth is indeed stranger than fiction." The names are of course fictitious, the physical descriptions and geographic locations have been changed to preserve anonymity.

Understanding how nutritional chemistry affects the mind has changed my life. Many patients have told me it changed theirs too. I think it is no exaggeration to claim that this book contains information which can change your life for the better.

This book is not, however, a self-help manual. This new field is immensely complicated; satisfactory treatment requires a good physician with a sound understanding of nutrition. Though I discuss cases in detail and give dosages for the education of practitioners, no two cases are alike. When employing treatment, always seek medical help.

I have written this book because I believe nutrition and vitamin therapy provides a safe, effective, and inexpensive therapeutic tool.

Nutrition
and
Vitamin Therapy

Nutrition and Vitamin Therapy

Let nothing which can be treated by diet be treated by other means.

MAIMONIDES (12th Century)

Nutrition and vitamin therapy applies the correct balance of substances normally in the body—vitamins, minerals, and other nutrients—and removes toxic molecules, such as lead, mercury, and cadmium.

We usually think when something is wrong with the mind, its cause is "mental." Most psychiatrists practice psychotherapy on the assumption that the problem is "all in the mind" and can be talked away. For much "mental" illness this is not the case. Whenever we have a feeling or thought, a chemical change must occur in the body. If we do not have the right chemicals present in the right amounts, our thoughts and feelings may be distorted. The brain, therefore, requires the proper chemicals obtained by good nutrition in order to work correctly. In fact, the brain is our most sensitive organ, reacting earlier to improper nutrition and the presence of toxins than any other system of the body.[1]

A Typical Case

The following case illustrates my method of practice. This patient, in contrast to the others cited throughout the book, is a fictional composite representing several typical problems.

Alan Jenson, a thirty-five-year-old dentist, enters my office. His shoulders are pulled in against his chest and his tightly clenched jaw juts forward.

"Leading with his chin," I think to myself, "the typical posture of the aggressive, ambitious Western male."

Alan's breathing is choked and shallow. His stooped-over posture suggests chronic depression. The raised shoulders and lack of movement of his frozen chest signal anxiety.

Alan's timid, squeezed voice sounds younger than his years. His fear-filled eyes seem alert for any sign of danger. His handshake is weak, hesitant, and cold. The hesitancy communicates a fearful, indecisive grasp on life. The coldness suggests anxiety and the constricted blood circulation of hypoglycemia (low blood sugar). The weak grasp implies fatigue, another symptom of depression and/or hypoglycemia. Alan slumps in his chair, a comfortable position for the chronically depressed, his back bowed from constant sorrow.

Alan tells me he is happily married, with two small children and a thriving practice. He would seem to have few problems; but clearly he is worried and unhappy.

"All my life," he relates, "I have been living for tomorrow. I can't remember the last time I was really happy. I guess I've been ambitious. In school I was always studying; I didn't have time to have fun. I was always living for this day when I would arrive—you know, married, raising a family, a house of my own, and a busy practice. Now I have it and I'm not happy," he sighs. "Is this it, is this what life has to offer? I planned everything so carefully, worked everything out to guarantee happiness. Now I have everything I'd planned for, but . . . it feels like something is missing."

"Something is missing?" I repeat, encouraging him to explore his feeling. I am, of course, also concerned with the social and psychological aspects of my patient's problems.

"Yes, I feel empty, I have an empty feeling, right here in the pit of my stomach."

"How long have you felt that way?" I inquire.

"As long as I can remember.... Actually, the first time was when I was about twelve. I was riding my bike near home, speeding very fast, racing away from our house, and as I was coasting I suddenly felt this gnawing emptiness in my stomach, like an ache. I guess maybe you could say it's loneliness."

"Who could say," I interjected, "me or you?"

"Huh, did I say you? I meant me, it's just a figure of speech," he replies, puzzled at my interruption.

"When describing yourself it's best if you stick to the first person. If it's *you* feeling something, say '*I* felt lonely.' It's *you* that's feeling it, right?

"But what about that empty feeling in the pit of your stomach?" I persist. "Do you feel it now?"

The young dentist looks thoughtful. "I guess you could say so."

"There you go again!" I respond.

"I mean yes, I do have that feeling. It's there all the time, but usually I don't notice it."

"Stand up, please," I ask. "Stand straight with your arms at your side." Even when he purposely stands straight, he retains his slouched posture. "Now please take off your shirt, lie down on my examining table, and point out where you have that empty feeling."

He places his finger on his stomach, in the center, just below his breast bone (sternum). I place my fingers on the spot he has identified and slowly, gently, I press in deep. I notice his breast bone has been pulled in on his stomach as the rectus abdominus, the muscle covering the abdomen, has been shortened by spasm.

"Ow! That's sore!" my patient exclaims.

"It hurts when I press because this muscle is in spasm. Just see if you can bear the pain while I try to press the spasm out." Using my hands like wedges, I press deeper on his abdominal muscle, moving very slowly to prevent the muscle from tightening against me. Suddenly, under my pressure, the spasm releases and the abdominal muscle lengthens.

"How does that feel now?" I ask.

"My stomach feels like a bowlful of jelly, all loose and quivery," he replies with awe, "and I feel *very* relaxed, as if I could fall asleep."

"Please don't, we still have work to do." He puts on his shirt and we resume our conversation.

"It's just that here I am, at the height of my powers, making good money, my wife is fine, my kids are great, and I should be happy. But I'm not. Instead, I dread going to work. I feel tired and exhausted. I get angry at the drop of a hat. Sometimes I cry for no reason and I just don't know what's wrong."

"Could you tell me about your diet?" I ask.

"What's my diet got to do with it?"

"It could have a lot to do with it. What you eat can affect the way you feel. Tell me what you have for breakfast."

"I don't usually have breakfast," Alan responds. "I start seeing patients at 8:00 A.M. and don't have time to eat. My nurse fixes coffee at the office, and sometimes she brings in doughnuts."

I try not to wince. "And then what?"

"I do take a long lunch," he continues. "Generally, I go over to Fuglio's on the corner and have pasta with French bread, maybe a few glasses of wine and an expresso. Then back to work. As soon as I get home I have a bourbon or two until dinner. Jean is an excellent cook. She puts a lot of variety into our dinners. Usually meat or fish, bread, potatoes, salads, coffee, and dessert. Her desserts are terrific. But I really don't think there's anything wrong with my diet," he protests as he points to his protruding abdomen. "As you can see, I get plenty to eat."

"It isn't the quantity I'm worried about, it's the quality. With all the coffee, alcohol, and rich starchy food you consume, low blood sugar could be responsible for your fatigue and depression."

During this first visit, I ask questions and look for specific signs to help me determine which tests may help me find the chemical imbalances responsible for my patient's difficulties.

New Kinds of Tests

"Your hands are cold," I tell him. "Are they often like that?"

"Yes, they are; my feet are cold too. Doesn't that mean my circulation is bad?"

"Maybe, but cold hands and feet are often symptoms of low blood sugar. I think we should order a blood sugar test."

"Oh, I just had one of those. My physician just gave me

a complete physical and did tests. He couldn't find anything wrong. That's why I came to you!"

"I don't mean a routine blood sugar. I'm talking about a *five-hour fasting glucose tolerance test.* Just a single blood sugar won't pick up hypoglycemia."

"A glucose tolerance test, how does that work?" Alan inquires.

"Eat nothing after midnight the night before. The morning of the test, remain fasting and go right to the lab. They draw a sample of blood to measure your fasting blood sugar. Then you drink a measured amount of sugar water and the lab takes hourly blood samples to see how your body handles sugar. During the test, observe how you feel. See if you get tired, weak, nervous, or sick in any way. Later we'll look at your blood sugar results and compare them with any symptoms you developed. If your blood sugar falls and you experience symptoms at the time of the drop, we call that hypoglycemia or low blood sugar. While you're at the laboratory we'll get some other blood and urine tests to check for possible biochemical imbalances causing your symptoms."

"What tests?"

"Let me see your fingernails. Look at those white spots. They may indicate a zinc deficiency. So we'll order a *blood zinc* and *copper level.*"

"Why the copper level?" asks Alan.

"Zinc is in balance with copper. To understand the significance of a blood zinc, we need a blood copper too. Let's also measure your *vitamin B_{12}* and *folic acid level.* These two B vitamins give us an idea of your B vitamin status; B vitamin deficiency can cause your symptoms. Do you suffer from any allergies?"

"I get 'hayfever' every spring."

"Please take a deep breath ... I notice you breathe through your mouth. Try breathing through your nose."

"I don't breathe easily through my nose. It's often clogged."

"Nasal stuffiness could be due to a chronic allergy. We can test the *blood histamine level.* Histamine causes the allergic reaction. So high histamine is a sign of allergy. Elevated histamine can cause depression, another reason to measure it.

"We can obtain a complete battery of *routine screening tests* which will indicate how well your organs and systems are working. The work is all automated, and these screening tests are inexpensive. Also, I'd like to obtain an analysis of your hair."

"My hair? What does that tell you?"

"The *hair analysis* measures the normal body *minerals*, such as calcium and magnesium, and also detects the presence of *toxic metals*, like lead and mercury. Because you're a dentist, mercury pollution is a real concern as your high-speed drill vaporizes the mercury amalgam and you may inhale toxic levels of mercury vapor."

"And too much mercury can make me depressed?"

"You've heard the expression 'mad as a hatter'? Mercury was used in the manufacture of felt hats, and it poisons the nerves and brain. Nervous symptoms are usually the first sign of mercury and other toxic metal poisons. So we definitely need to analyze your hair for heavy metals. It will take a few weeks to collect all the test results. While we're waiting, would you please record everything you eat for a week? I don't care what you eat, but be truthful and complete. Bring it with you at our next visit."

"O.K. Thanks. Oh, how do I do the hair analysis?"

"Clip about two heaping tablespoons of hair, put it in an envelope, and send it to this laboratory. Since this is your first hair analysis, you can use the ends of your hair. Just give yourself a trim. Later if we want to check the hair again, we take hair close to the scalp because we want the new hair which will reflect recent changes."

The Results of Alan's Blood Sugar Test

Three weeks later we meet again. I ask Alan about his experience with the glucose tolerance test.

"The morning of the test I had a slight headache, but after they gave me the sugar drink I was fine. Two hours later, however, I felt very weak. I got a splitting headache and stomach cramps. My eyes blurred and I became jittery, irritable, and depressed. Then I became very drowsy and fell asleep. By the fourth hour I felt a little better. After the test was over, I still felt very weak and famished. I went out and ate and felt a little better. But I was miserable for the next forty-eight hours. That's quite a test!"

Alan's blood sugar curve (Figure 1) shows that the first fasting blood sugar was 90 mg % (90 milligrams of glucose sugar in 100 milliliters of blood), which is normal. After the glucose drink, it peaked to 150 mg % and Alan felt fine. But then his blood sugar plummeted to 40 mg % by the third hour, and simultaneously he felt "terrible, irritable, and depressed." This sudden reactive drop in blood sugar coupled with symptoms at the time of the drop is called low blood sugar or hypoglycemia.

FIGURE 1

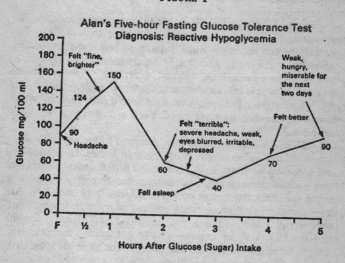

Alan's Five-hour Fasting Glucose Tolerance Test
Diagnosis: Reactive Hypoglycemia

Low blood sugar affects the entire body, but especially the brain which can only burn sugar and uses 25% of all the food we eat. Brain sugar starvation can cause splitting headaches, blurred vision, and depression.

The drop in blood sugar even caused Alan to fall asleep, probably a protective reaction. A horizontal sleeping position makes it easier for the body to keep the brain bathed in blood.

The diagnosis is *reactive* hypoglycemia because Alan's first fasting blood sugar was normal, becoming low only *in reaction* to taking sugar.

Alan's headache before the test could mean his overnight fast had precipitated a withdrawal symptom from a food addiction.

How I Use Alan's Dietary Record

Alan's weekly dietary record gives me a clue to his food addiction.

Alan drinks several cups of coffee throughout the day. Coffee is a very common food addiction, perhaps the most common. Something like 90% of the adult population drinks coffee daily.

When I raised this issue with the young dentist, he protested: "But I *need* the morning coffee to wake up. I'm completely out of sorts until I have a few cups of coffee. Please don't ask me to give it up!" he groaned.

"Spoken like a true addict," I replied. "You're caught in a vicious cycle. Coffee addiction is aggravating your low blood sugar, but you can only avoid the pain of withdrawal by having another cup. You're a prisoner of your addiction."

"Then I'm a prisoner of love, because I love my coffee!"

"Coffee's a diuretic, causing vitamin losses. In particular, coffee causes a vitamin B_1 (thiamine) deficiency which, in turn, causes nervousness and depression, the very symptoms you're suffering from. But coffee is not the only problem. All the sugars and refined starches you eat may be upsetting your mood too," I said. "These rich desserts: soft drinks, doughnuts, cookies, and ice cream—you've got quite a sweet tooth! Also, look at all the refined starches. French bread, spaghetti, pizza—and alcohol. Alcohol is rapidly absorbed into the bloodstream and causes the same blood sugar roller-coaster ride. Here's a hypoglycemia diet. Please avoid foods on the avoid list and choose your foods only from the foods allowed." (See Figure 2.)

Alan studies the diet, looks thoughtful, and says, "This is going to cause Jean a problem. She'll have to cook separately for me."

"Put the whole family on this diet," I replied. "Dr. Cheraskin studied blood sugar in spouses and found husbands and wives have remarkably similar blood sugar curves—perhaps because they eat the same foods, or it may be that people are attracted to mates with similar chemical makeups.

The term 'chemical attraction' could be more true than we realize.

"Add more protein and complex carbohydrates. By complex carbohydrates I mean legumes, whole fruits, and vegetables. These foods take longer to digest, break down to sugar slowly, and, therefore, don't stimulate a big insulin response. Avoid simple carbohydrates, such as white sugar and white flour products which enter the bloodstream quickly and provoke a severe insulin response. You eat only two or three times a day. Try eating smaller meals more frequently; eat six or seven times a day. It's best if you never feel hungry. If you eat every three hours your blood sugar will never dip low enough to cause symptoms."

I also advise Alan to get regular physical exercise, which is usually beneficial to hypoglycemics. By improving the circulation and breathing, and toning up the muscles, exercise improves the function of cellular metabolism. Further, physical exercise moves blood sugar into the body's cells without requiring insulin. This sparing of insulin release prevents the reactive drop in blood sugar.

Note the excessively high calcium and magnesium and abnormally low sodium and potassium levels in Alan's hair analysis (see Figure 3). This is a characterstic pattern seen in low blood sugar out of control.

The hair analysis also reveals elevated levels of the toxic metals lead, cadmium, and mercury.

The mercury could come from his work with the high-speed dentist's drill. Mercury is also concentrated in big fish, like tuna, which the diet sheet indicates he eats frequently. Small fish, like sardines, are less polluted with mercury and thus safer. The lead is probably from air pollution. Most city dwellers have high lead levels.

The low levels of iron, chromium, and zinc in Alan's hair mean he's probably not getting enough of these normal minerals in his diet. A body starved for the normal metals will pick up heavy metals in their place and attempt to use them in its chemical reactions. Using the heavy metals, rather than the normal ones, gums up the works. Adding more meats and vegetables to his diet and eating only unprocessed foods will increase his normal mineral content, lowering his susceptibility to heavy metal pollution.

The high cadmium level probably comes from his two packs a day of cigarettes.

FIGURE 2

A HYPOGLYCEMIC DIET

Abbreviations: C = Carbohydrate, P = Protein, F = Fat. The numbers are the approximate percentages of Carbohydrate (C), Protein (P), and Fat (F) in the particular food.

FOODS TO AVOID	C	P	F		C	P	F
Refined (white) sugar; and all foods containing refined sugar	100	—	—	Maraschino cherry	50	—	—
				Gelatin powder	35	—	—
Refined (white) flour; and all foods made from it, such as				Marmalade	65	—	—
				Commercial ice cream	20	4	13
Crackers	72	9	9	Coffee	.8	.3	.1
Cake, cookies	65	6	9	Jelly with white sugar	70	—	—
Noodles, spaghetti, macaroni	19	4	—	Unsweetened dry cocoa	38	18	20
Doughnuts	52	7	22	Sweet chocolate	60	2	25
Wheat or rye refined bread	50	9	3	Tapioca pudding	28	3	3
Refined cereals	77	11	1	Catsup	24	2	—
Refined (white) rice	24	3	—				

FOODS TO EAT SPARINGLY							
Honey	81	—	—	Dried fruits, such as			
Crude brown sugar	91	.4	.5	Dates	78	2	3
Maple syrup, molasses	65	—	—	Figs	68	4	—
Fruit juice (orange & grapefruit are best tolerated)				Prunes	65	2	—
				Sweet potato	19	2	1
Orange juice, fresh	10.4	.7	.2	Potato chips	49	7	37
Grape juice	19	—	—	Popcorn	80	12	5
Prune juice	18	—	—	Fresh dates	65	2	—
Apple juice	13	—	—	Potato	17	2	.1
Baked beans	19	6	2	Corn	19	3	1
Black tea	.4	.1	—	Prepared coconut	50	4	39

FOODS ALLOWED							
Cherries	17	1	1	Grapefruit	10	—	—
Parsnips	16	2	1	Peaches	10	1	—
Grapes	15	1	1	Orange	13	—	—
Blueberries	15	1	1	Mulberries	13	—	—
Lentils	57	25	1	Blackberries	12	1	1
Lima Beans	15	4	—	Lemon	8	1	—
Salad Dressing	15	5	10	Root Beet	9	2	—
Apple	14	—	—	White Onion	9	2	—
Pineapple	14	—	—	Green Peas	9	4	—
Red Peppers	7	1	1	Yeast	8	8	—
Winter Squash	7	1	—	Carrots	8	1	—
Watermelon	6	—	—	Cauliflower	2	1	—
Fresh Soybeans	6	13	7	Cucumber	2	1	—
Pumpkin	6	1	—	Lettuce	2	1	—
Clams	.5	11	1	Spinach	2	1	—
Oysters	5	8	1	Watercress	2	1	—
Cantaloupe	5	1	—	Pickles, Sour, Dill	2	—	—
Kale	5	2	—	American Cheese	2	27	32

FOODS ALLOWED	C	P	F		C	P	F
Turnip Beet, Green	5	1	—	Cream Cheese	2	7	34
Custard	5	6	7	Other Cheese	2	20	32
Whole Milk	5	4	4	Eggplant	18	5	1
Skimmed Milk	5	4	—	Bean Sprouts	26	16	1
Buttermilk	5	4	.1	Mushrooms	1	1	—
Light Cream	5	4	12	All Meat Frankfurter	1	19	18
Average Cream	5	3	19	Butter	—	1	81
Brussel Sprouts	4	1	19	Whole Egg	1	13	12
Vinegar	4	—	—	Egg White	—	1	—
Creamed Soup	4	2	13	Egg Yolk	—	16	30
Tomatoes	4	1	—	Sardines, Canned	—	23	20
Green Pepper	4	1	—	Herring, Smoked	—	37	16
Eggplant	4	1	—	Salmon	—	21	12
Cabbage	4	1	—	Other Fish	—	19	8
Broccoli	4	3	—	Halibut	—	18	6
Green Beet	4	2	—	Herring	—	20	7
Cottage Cheese	4	20	1	Bass	—	20	2
Heavy Cream	3	2	41	Cod	—	20	1
Summer Squash	3	1	—	Tuna Fish	3	2	2
Sauerkraut	3	1	—	Lean Broiled Beef	—	28	5
Rhubarb	3	1	—	Chicken or Duck	—	21	5
Radishes	3	1	—	Peanut Butter	3	4	7
Celery	3	1	—	Kidney	—	16	6
String Beans	3	1	—	Liver	—	20	5
Asparagus	3	1	—	Medium fat Veal	—	20	11
Artichokes, French	3	1	—	Lamb or Mutton	—	19	15
Scallops	3	15	—	Tongue	—	16	15
Avocado	3	2	26	Fat, Med. Done Beef	—	13	18
Ripe or Green Olives	3	2	15	Beef Heart	—	16	20
Fresh, lean Ham	—	25	14	Lamb Chops	—	20	22
Turkey	—	22	18	Cod Liver Oil	—	—	100
Chick Peas	12	4	1	Cooking Fat	—	—	100
All Meat Sausage	—	18	38	Lard or Shortening	—	—	100
Mayonnaise	—	2	75	Salad and Cooking Oils	—	—	100
Banana	22	1	—	Limes	13	—	—
Miscellaneous nuts	20	2	60	Fresh Apricots	13	1	—
Fresh Prunes	19	1	—	Applesauce	13	—	—
Fresh Figs	18	1	—	Cranberries	10	1	1
Persimmons	18	1	—	Dry Soybeans	34	34	18
Fresh Plums	12	1	—	Raspberries	12	1	1

To plan your diet, you need not use these food lists. Simply avoid all refined foods (white sugar, white flour, white rice, pasta), jam and jelly, ice cream, cocoa, alcoholic beverages, cola and soft drinks, strong black tea and coffee. It may be possible to have one or two cups of coffee daily, but only after eating a meal.

Narcotics, stimulants, and depressant drugs should be avoided. Artificial sweeteners are not recommended for other reasons. Salt is permitted, especially during hot weather.

Especially preferred are meat, fish, fowl, eggs, dairy, and vegetables. It is important to eat between meals and before retiring. Nutritional supplements (brewer's yeast, dessicated liver, multivitamins) are often desirable. Lengthly daily exercise is important.

Whenever possible, eat only fresh foods. Frozen and canned foods should be avoided or used sparingly because of their reduced content of nutrients.

"Cadmium is used in processing, along with several other chemicals, and, of course, sugar," I inform Alan.

"Sugar too?"

"You've heard of sugar-cured tobacco? Tobacco has been implicated in everything from heart disease to cancer. If you can't quit altogether, then switch to a natural cigarette, containing only tobacco, and try to smoke less."

"Now I know why you're Dr. Lesser," he replied with a grim smile. "You want me to eat less sugar, drink less coffee and alcohol, smoke less. I was depressed before I came here. You want to take away the little pleasure in life I still have."

"Cadmium in small quantitites has been implicated in heart disease. A good way to lower that hair cadmium level is to stop smoking commercial cigarettes. It's best, of course, to just stop smoking."

"Well, what about the lead, mercury, and cadmium I've got now?" inquired Alan. "How do I get rid of what I already have?"

"We can remove those with 'chelators' which chemically bond with the heavy metal and pull it out of the body. Beans and eggs contain natural chelators, sulfhydryl groups, composed of sulfur and hydrogen molecules. The pectin in applesauce is also helpful. The amino acids cystine and methionine also contain sulfhydryl groups and chelate heavy metals. Vitamin C is also a chelator. It also enhances the absorption of some minerals from food.

"There are some other findings in your blood tests which may have a bearing on your problem. Your serum copper is 165 mg % and your serum zinc is only 95 mg %. That is an improper balance."

"What does it mean?"

"It means you have either too much copper or not enough zinc. The body (and mind) is in optimal balance when there are ten parts zinc to nine parts copper. In your case, the copper level is much too high relative to zinc. An excessive copper/zinc ratio may be responsible for your symptoms. Excessive copper can cause depression, irritability, alienation, anger, and even paranoia."

"Where could I be getting all that copper?" he asked.

"How old is your house?" I inquired.

"We have a new house, had it built ourselves."

"Then most likely you have copper plumbing. Our city water is slightly acid. When that acid water sits in the copper pipes at night, some copper goes into the water. Your excess copper may be coming from your drinking water. Let your water run in the morning so you don't drink the water which has stood in the pipes overnight. You can also absorb significant copper from your cookware. Some of the most widely sold multivitamin formulas contain 2 mg of copper, which is excessive. Elevated blood copper appears to be quite common; I find twenty high serum copper levels for every one that is low."

"What about the extra copper already in me?" inquired Alan. "How do we get rid of that?"

"A simple and safe way is to prescribe zinc. Zinc has an inverse relationship to cooper: as we raise your blood zinc, that will lower your blood copper."

The Fundamental Level

"All right, I'm going to make the changes in my diet, take the supplements you suggest, get more exercise, and watch my posture. But this is very different from what I expected. I expected you'd find my problems were psychological."

"Human behavior is complicated. Health consists of maintaining a balance on many levels. No obvious imbalance in your psychological health is apparent. You're happy with your relationships, you enjoy your work, or did before you became depressed. The chemical molecular level is the fundamental level. In examining your chemistry, we've found several instances of imbalance. All our efforts now are directed at restoring your molecular balance. If the diet and supplements don't help, then, of course, we'll look more deeply at other levels."

Alan underwent a few days of unpleasant withdrawal from coffee, alcohol, and cigarettes, experiencing headaches and sore muscles. But then he felt a lot better and had more energy. After four weeks, the excessive copper cleared from his body, and he experienced a lifting of his depression.

Alan studied yoga to improve his breathing and posture. With the addition of psychotherapy, he began to change his "driven" life style. Several months later he was feeling better and happier than ever before in his life.

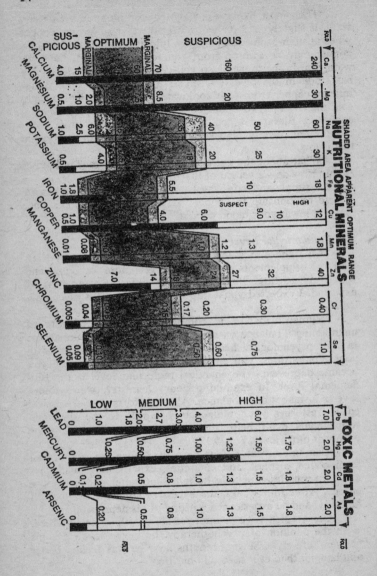

FIGURE 3

Alan's Hair Analysis

MineraLab, Inc.
3046 ... Court, Fremont, CA 94538 · 415/489-5535
46 MASSACHUSETTS Avenue, Boston, MA 01776 617/266-2716

HAIR ANALYSIS REPORT

PERSONAL INFORMATION

NAME: JENSON, ALAN

Sex   M
Age   35   Hair Location   Head
Ht.   5' 11"   Hair Color, NATURAL Blonde
Wt.   178 lb.   Hair Coloring None.
Race   Cauc. Shampoo ———
                Occupation Dentist

RETURN
TO
ADDRESS

BATCH - SAMPLE
CONTROL-NO.
DATE REC'D.
DATE COMPLETED

SIGNIFICANT RATIOS

MINERALS	VALUE	MIDLINE IDEAL
Ca: Mg		8:1
Ca: Mn		80:1
Ca: Zn		2:1
Na: K		2:1
Fe: Cu		1.5:1
Zn: Cu		8:1
Zn: Mn		40:1
Zn: Cd		2000:1
Zn: Pb		200:1

NOTE: ALL MINERALS REPORTED IN mg%
(1 mg% = 10 ppm)

This case illustrates how nutrition and vitamin therapy works. First, we gather a history, including dietary information gained by asking the patient to record a week's diet. Physical examination often reveals clues as to possible biochemical imbalances. Laboratory studies reveal how well the body's organs and systems work. We also measure the patient's actual vitamin and mineral levels and check the level of heavy metal pollutants.

Nutrition and vitamin therapy consists of balancing the body's chemicals: increasing those that are deficient, decreasing those that are excessive, and removing those not naturally present in the body, such as the heavy metals.

2

A Brief History of Nutrition and Vitamin Therapy

The Discovery of Vitamins

From ancient times, it was a widely held folk belief that fresh foods contained necessary elements to prevent disease and promote health. The Black Death of the fourteenth century killed millions of Crusaders and city dwellers in Europe. This plague was perhaps due as much to the lack of fresh food and the resulting nutritional deficiencies as to the actual infectious bacteria. Persons living in the countryside with access to fresh food had greater resistance and remained largely unaffected.

The crucial experiment proving fresh food contained an element which prevented scurvy (a vitamin C deficiency which causes weakness, disease, and death) was performed by James Lind in 1747. Lind, surgeon's mate of the H.M.S. *Salisbury*, divided twelve seamen suffering similar degrees of survy into six pairs. Each pair's regular diet was supplemented with a commonly used treatment for scurvy. One pair was fed a quart of cider daily, a second received twenty-five drops of dilute sulfuric acid three times daily, the third pair was given two spoonfuls of vinegar three times daily, the

17

fourth half a pint of sea water three times a day, the fifth a concoction of herbs, and the sixth received two oranges and one lemon daily for six days. the last pair recovered so rapidly they were used as nurses for the others. There was slight improvement in the cider pair but none at all in the others.

This was definitive evidence that citrus fruits cured scurvy. Although Lind didn't realize it, he had found a good natural source of vitamin C.

Not until 1795 did the British Admiralty officially adopt Lind's simple preventive measure of an ounce of lemon juice per man. This wiped out scurvy in the English navy, securing their dominance of the high seas. English naval officers of the time asserted it was equivalent to doubling their fighting force, soon dubbed "limeys."

Though it was now known that fresh food could prevent scurvy, it was disputed whether scurvy was caused by the absence of certain constituents in the food or by the presence of an actual poison.

In the early nineteenth century, experiments were conducted in which animals were fed purified diets of the then-known food constituents: fats, carbohydrates, and proteins. The animals did not grow and developed an opacity of the cornea of the eye (which we now know is due to a vitamin A deficiency).

Why a purified diet, adequate in proteins, carbohydrates, and fats, would not support life remained a mystery throughout the nineteenth century. But this experiment hinted that food must contain other factors besides proteins, carbohydrates, and fats in order to sustain life.

In 1830, Muller in Switzerland built the steel-roller wheat mill, and the use of refined flour spread throughout Europe and the other industrialized nations. The use of refined sugar paralleled this spread. With the advent of these refined foods (white flour, white rice, and white sugar), vitamin deficiency diseases became widespread. One of these illnesses, beriberi, affected 25 to 40% of the Imperial Japanese fleet.

Beriberi, caused by a lack of vitamin B_1, is characterized by numbness and paralysis of the legs and arms and leads to cardiac and respiratory distress and death. In 1882, Director-General of the Japanese Medical Service, Kanehiro Takaki,[1] cured beriberi by decreasing the ration of polished white rice and increasing the use of whole barley, vegetables, meat, and milk. But Takaki didn't understand that the better diet was supplying a missing food factor; he believed the cure was due to the higher caloric intake.

In 1886 a young Dutch physician, Christiaan Eijkman, assigned to study beriberi, noticed that chickens in the laboratory chickenhouse were dying of a paralytic disease closely resembling beriberi. While Eijkman was studying the chickens' disease, those that had not died mysteriously recovered and no new cases developed. Investigating, he found the chickens had been fed polished (white) rice, prepared in the military hospital kitchen for the hospital patients. When a new cook took charge of the kitchen, he refused to "allow military rice for civilian chickens." From that point on, when the chickens were returned to coarse unpolished (brown) rice, the chickens' paralytic disease and deaths ceased. Eijkman immediately confirmed that a diet of polished rice caused death in three or four weeks, whereas the chickens remained in good health when fed unpolished rice.

Eijkman went on to determine in a study of 200,000 Dutch West Indies prisoners that the incidence of beriberi was 300 times as great in prisons where polished rice was a staple of the diet, as in those where unpolished rice was used. By 1907, Eijkman had concluded that the bran of the rice contained a nutrient substance required for good health.

Awareness of the importance of minerals in living systems began a little earlier, in 1820, when the Geneva physician Coindet reported the highly successful treatment of simple goiter using iodine.[2] As recently as fifty years ago, the only minerals recognized as essential for healthy function were iodine and iron; we now know of eight or ten minerals that are important.

In 1911, Polish scientist Casimir Funk[3] first proposed that there were antiscurvy, antiberiberi, antipellagra, and antirickets factors in foods. He called these food factors "vitamines," from the Latin word *vita* (life) and the chemical term amine, a member of a class of compounds of nitrogen. When it was later found that not all essential food factors contain nitrogen, the name was changed to vitamin.

In the first quarter of this century, many scientists set to work to isolate and identify just what these "vitamines" were. To do this, it was necessary to concentrate the substance from natural extracts, isolate it in pure form, and crystalize and recrystallize it to ensure it was one single chemical compound. Only then could it be chemically identified and its molecular structure determined.

In 1928, Budapest-born Albert Szent-Györgyi succeeded in isolating crystals of a sugarlike substance from the adrenal gland of the ox. He determined the chemical formula of the substance to be $C_6H_8O_6$ (six carbon and oxygen atoms and eight hydrogen atoms). He gave some of the crystalline material to W. N. Haworth, the English sugar chemist, who found its structural formula. Szent-Györgyi and Haworth named the substance ascorbic acid, meaning the acidic substance that prevents scurvy. In 1937, these two chemists received the Nobel Prize for their discovery and synthesis of ascorbic acid, vitamin C.

Within a short time ascorbic acid became available in drug stores and food stores, but for many years it was believed that the amount of this vitamin and the other newly discovered vitamins necessary for good health was only the amount required to prevent outright disease and death.

Pioneers of Vitamin Therapy

A few physicians decided to try substantial amounts of these recently isolated vitamin and mineral nutrients to test their effectiveness against diseases for which there was no known remedy. None of these pioneers did their work at large renowned academic centers; they were all clinicians with their own practices or working in out-of-the-way hospitals.

In the 1940s, Dr. William Kaufman[4] in his Connecticut private practice found that high doses of nicotinamide, a B vitamin, effectively reversed arthritis. In 1948, Dr. Frederick Klenner,[5] a physician in a small town in Virginia, published the first in a series of twenty-eight papers documenting his conclusion that "when the proper amounts (of vitamin C) are used it will destroy all virus organisms." Dr. Klenner wiped out viral diseases ranging from simple cold sores to hepatitis of the liver by giving intravenous or intramuscular injections ranging from 30 to 100 g of vitamin C (30,000 to 100,000 mg) a day. In 1949, working in a small hospital in Australia, psychiatrist John F. Cade[6] discovered megadoses of lithium, a mineral, would quiet manic patients; and in 1952, Drs. Abram Hoffer and Humphrey Osmond[7] first announced in Saskatoon, Saskatchewan Province, Canada, that megadoses of nicotinamide and vitamin C, together with a high protein diet, helped schizophrenics.

Hoffer and Osmond's first case was a young farm boy, lapsed into a catatonic stupor, unable to talk, eat, or use the bathroom. He did not respond to insulin or electric shock, the best available treatments at the time, and steadily deteriorated. Finally the boy's family was notified he would die. The boy was in coma, with death approaching, when in desperation Drs. Hoffer and Osmond fed him 10 g of niacin and 5 g of vitamin C through a stomach tube. Two days later the boy was out of coma and able to take the vitamins himself in a glass of water. Two weeks later he was normal. He remains so to this day, now a married man, owner of a prosperous construction firm.

The work of these pioneers aroused little interest in the medical community because the "miracle drugs" were commanding all the attention. Newly introduced antibiotics, tranquilizers, and steroids acted quickly and seemed highly effective. Drug companies, which held exclusive patents on these chemicals, spent millions on promotion and further research into so-called wonder drugs. Nutrients, being natural substances, could not be patented; and since drug companies couldn't hold patents on nutrients, they lacked incentive for researching and promoting nutrient therapies.

In 1968, Dr. Linus Pauling defined orthomolecular psychiatry as the achievement and preservation of mental health by varying the concentrations in the human body of substances that are normally present, such as the vitamins. This definition greatly clarified and crystalized the emerging therapy. Winner of the Nobel Prize in Chemistry (1954) and the Nobel Peace Prize (1963), Dr. Pauling was widely known and highly regarded; his personal prestige added weight to the idea that large orthomolecular doses of nutrients might be effective against disease.

A Brief Autobiography

I Discover Freud

In 1955, when I was sixteen and living in my hometown of Mitchell, South Dakota, I hastily devoured a tunafish sandwich and rushed out to see a friend. Suddenly I was choking and gasping for breath. I fell to the ground, frightened I would die. Mercifully, the attack passed in a half-minute. Two days later, I experienced a second choking spasm and in another two days a third, this time at home, in front of my family. Our family physician rushed me to the hospital. I had three more attacks in the hospital, all while I was asleep, and then they stopped.

After I returned home, my father sent me to the doctor's office to find out why our health insurance had not paid for my hospitalization. The doctor had diagnosed my condition as hysteria and the insurance didn't cover nervous illness. Not knowing what hysteria was, at the Public Library I found a reference to Dr. Sigmund Freud. The library carried a worn and tattered copy of his *Three Essays on a Theory of Sexuality*. The book fascinated me, and I subsequently read everything of Freud's I could find.

Freud related everything to sex, which seemed to fit the inclinations of my sixteen-year-old body. Freud's writings suggested that my plan to be an artist was only a sublimation of sexual desire. I lost interest in art and developed interest in girls. I also decided to imitate my new idol by becoming a doctor and psychoanalyst like him.

In and Out of the Ivory Tower

Studying at Cornell University Medical College, New York City, in 1962, I worked for Peter Stokes, well-known endocrinologist of the New York Hospital Payne Whitney Psychiatric Clinic. We researched mood and cortisol, the main hormone of the cortex of the adrenal gland. We found that when patients are anxious or depressed, their blood cortisol rose, and when they were in an elated euphoric state, cortisol dropped, a clear enunciation of the inseparable connection between mental states and the adrenal hormones.[8]

After graduating from medical school in 1964, I interned at the Upstate Medical Center in Syracuse where the famous Hungarian psychoanalyst Thomas Szasz, author of *The Myth of Mental Illness*, taught. Szasz believes mental illness isn't an "illness" at all, but what is called illness is really just social behavior deviating from the usual. Psychiatrists, he feels, function as unwitting keepers of the social order. By labeling people "mentally ill" and committing them to locked institutions, society deprives psychiatric patients of their civil rights, when their only "crime" is social deviancy.

While I was at Syracuse, the English psychiatrist R. D.

Laing visited upstate New York. Like Szasz, Laing views the psychotic as a social deviant, one for whom insanity is a valid voyage of discovery. For Laing, there is nothing "wrong" with psychotics. Their behavior is understandable and, in fact, the only possible way of dealing with their particular family and society.

For my residency in psychiatry I returned to New York City to the Albert Einstein Medical Center, Jacobi Hospital in the Bronx. Laing, Szasz, and other social psychiatrists were very much in vogue, reflecting the general social concern of the sixties.

In accordance with these social theories of mental illness, the psychotic was seen as a sort of Cinderella who was the scapegoat of "sick" families. Gregory Bateson's "double-bind" theory, which held that psychotics were literally driven mad by their families, was popular. These people were the "Jesus Christ" martyrs whose madness was the price to be paid for keeping the rest of the family functional. The psychotic's mother was considered particularly guilty, called "schizophrenogenic." The patient himself was not to blame. His "illness" was due to victimization by his family and society in general. Neurotics, psychotics, drug addicts, alcoholics, sexual perverts, and delinquents were not responsible. They weren't "sick." They were socially deviant, forced to be so by bad mothering and social injustice. Treatment therefore, consisted of helping the patient win his "rights," or of treating the "sick family," or of creating social justice. Psychotherapy sought to understand the anger of the psychotic as justifiable rebellion against a sick society and tyrannical parents.

The Einstein Medical Center was a bastion of this view of mental illness as well as a haven for the older Freudian focus on the individual's psychological dynamics. Biochemical treatments were slowly gaining currency, fueled by the undeniable ability of the chemical tranquilizers to "cure" mental illness.

However, failure seemed to doom all these approaches. Psychotics would receive psychotherapy for an hour a day, five days a week for six months. In the protected hospital environment they would pull themselves together enough to be discharged. But at the first incidental stress of the outside world, they returned to the hospital, as psychotic as before, their understanding of the unconscious psychological dynamics of their illness providing no apparent help. Similarly, family therapy with patients and their families would continue sometimes for years. In the end, the patient was still unable to function, the blame laid on the family's unwillingness to "let go." Chemical tranquilizers were usually effective in the short term but kept most patients so drugged they couldn't function. The tranquilizers' side effects were so unpleasant that patients often stopped taking them and promptly relapsed. Even when the patient continued on drugs, at some completely unpredictable point the dragon of psychosis would rear its head and the patient would relapse anyway. The tranquilizers also presented a new danger; they often caused depression as a side effect. Not a few patients committed suicide by taking overdoses of their prescribed medication.

While a psychiatric resident at Einstein, I first heard of Hoffer and Osmond's megavitamin therapy from the desperate family of a patient. I was the fourth doctor to treat this pitiful young woman, an appealing but hopeless case.

When I mentioned the family's suggestion of megavitamin therapy to my supervisor, he dismissed the treatment as ineffective and wondered if the family weren't trying to sabotage our efforts by even bringing up the idea.

Completing my psychiatric residency in 1968, I then served two years in the U.S. Public Health Service. I was assigned to direct a narcotic addiction rehabilitation program at Terminal Island Prison in Long Beach, California. Life for me in the prison wasn't too tough because, unlike the inmates, I got to go home at night. The prisoners were friendlier than mental patients had been, and the experience contributed greatly to my education. I'd worked in hospitals with those whom society considered mad; now I was discovering those whom it called bad.

My views on human nature were gradually evolving. Since first reading Freud, I'd been fascinated with individual psychology. In psychoanalytic psychotherapy, the effort was to uncover the patient's past conflicts and, by making significant interpretations, help him break free of the old neurotic pattern. But I felt the main improvement came from the corrective *relationship* between the patient and the therapist and not from any understanding of his case the patient obtained. When the therapist makes an interpretation, not only is he giving information, he is also showing an *interest* in his patient. The most "therapeutic" part of analysis seems not so much what is learned but rather that another authoritative human being is *interested*. But psychotherapy was slow and uncertain, working on educated, introspective intellectuals. Fine for a portion of the population: what about the rest?

Understanding the importance of the relationship helped me appreciate Eric Berne (*Games People Play*) and Transactional Analysis, which focuses on the types of relationships between people.

Putting relationship therapy into practice at Terminal Island, we employed group therapy, turning the addicts' prison dormitory into a therapeutic community as described by John Cummings and Maxwell Jones.[9] Addicts appeared to be shy, alienated people, frightened of life, seeking an escape. My program was coeducational; many of the women had supported their drug habits by prostitution. But though they had slept with the opposite sex, they'd never *talked* to them. Group therapy was for most of the addicts their first exposure to an intimate social relationship with others. We held mass community meetings, marathon meetings which lasted two to three days, group meetings, dorm meetings, family sessions, and special groups, such as the "low riders" group for Mexican-American "Chicanos." This provided a new outlet for their energy and reduced the need to fix. But the social level also had its limitations. A few of the addicts even cracked up from the enforced intimacy of constant grouping.

Schizophrenia Must Be a Chemical Disorder

At that time volunteering at the Hollywood Free Clinic, I treated many users of psychedelic drugs who experienced "bum trips." Their bum trips were so similar in appearance to acute schizophrenia that I reasoned schizophrenia must be a chemical disorder. If a tiny amount of a chemical could cause temporary insanity in a previously normal person, perhaps psychotics were suffering the effects of a toxic chemical produced within their own systems. The psychotic was his own drug-abuse factory, doomed to a trip he could never end.

The actual core of schizophrenia, the altered perception of reality, couldn't be psychological; it had to be chemically induced. Mental delusions, confusion, inability to concentrate, hallucinations, and other distortions of perception were all predictable consequences of a chemically imbalanced brain presenting an altered picture of reality. Of course, a chemically imbalanced brain would express itself with altered perceptions of sight (visual hallucinations), sound (auditory hallucinations), taste ("food tastes strange," "my food is poisoned"), proprioception ("spiders are crawling on my skin"), and so on. I understood why talk therapy for schizophrenia had been like trying to stop a tank with a water pistol, and I saw why the vitamins might help. The schizophrenic manufactures his own LSD, and the vitamins help "soak up" and detoxify the hallucinogenic chemicals. Later, one schizophrenic even complained that since he'd been taking the B vitamin niacin and vitamin C he couldn't "get off" on LSD any more. Whenever he wanted to "trip" on psychedelics, he had to stop the vitamins for a few days.

Treating one bum tripper with Thorazine at the Free Clinic helped me understand why schizophrenics complain so bitterly about the phenothiazine tranquilizer's side effects. As the thoughtful and intelligent drug user, a medical student, explained after he had "come down," the cure was almost worse than the disease.

"The tranquilizer brought me down all right, and I'm grateful for that, but it wrenched me down," he related. "The side effects were most unpleasant, drying my mouth and making my tongue thick so my speech was slurred. The drug also caused restlessness; I couldn't sit still and paced about, out of control. The worst effect was on my brain. I couldn't think clearly, couldn't form a cogent thought, as if a dybbuk were strangling my mind. The drug made me drowsy, forcing me to bed to try to sleep off the effects."

After that I used only mild tranquilizers, like Valium or Librium, to treat bad drug trips, and often prescribed nothing, simply talking the patient down. In many cases psychotics benefited as much from mild tranquilizers as they had from the major drugs, and thereby avoided side effects.

As my Public Health Service duty drew to a close, I received a case in my small outside practice destined to add a revolutionary dimension to my understanding of human nature, and to thoroughly shatter many of the psychological theories I held so uneasily.

My First Two Nutrition and Vitamin Therapy Cases

Robert had cracked up at age eighteen in his first year at college. He wrote lengthy, bizarre letters home, signing them

"Jonathan Hell." Hospitalized for four and a half years, Robert received electroshock therapy, sedatives, and group psychotherapy in a vain effort to interrupt his malignant disease. He was "uncooperative," running away from the hospital whenever he could. Finally Robert was judged incurable, and the hospital superintendent recommended a prefrontal lobotomy. Widely used for "disturbed" schizophrenics in the early 1950s, the operation consisted of entering the skull above the eye and severing the connections betwen the thinking part (cerebral cortex) and the feeling part (thalamus) of the brain. This surgery turned raging troubled souls into docile vegetables, which in the eyes of many constituted a cure. Robert's family refused the surgery, so he was discharged to their care, living at home for twenty years.

Now forty-three, Robert continued to be beset by furies. He heard malevolent voices which tormented and criticized him continuously. In his more lucid periods, he wrote or phoned the FBI asking for J. Edgar Hoover, to warn him of vague nefarious plots, of which Robert was the inevitable victim. Usually he was too withdrawn to care. He showed no concern for his appearance, didn't bathe, and ate only if food were prepared and presented to him. He never left his inner world of madness long enough to concentrate on any activity. Robert was unable to work, read, or watch television. Often distraught, he would run away, only to be quickly picked up by the police and returned home. He smoked constantly and his fingers were nicotine-stained and scarred. With psychotic indifference, he frequently allowed the cigarette to burn until it singed his hand.

Unshaven, unkempt, laughing to himself, he engaged in a mumbling dialogue with the voices: "Nothing refers to nothing," he would respond to my questions; "I'm making no contracts!" he screamed apprehensively.

Such was Robert's state when his exhausted family brought him in, requesting I try megavitamin therapy. I was skeptical; the idea of taking a cetain diet and vitamins to treat mental illness seemed farfetched. But the past few years I'd taken a B vitamin complex myself, which seemed to increase my endurance and make me calmer and better able to handle stress. My wife had interested me in nutrition and I'd read Adelle Davis.

The megavitamin pioneer, Humphrey Osmond, was now

working at the University of Alabama, and I phoned him to discuss the advisability of the nutrient therapy in Robert's case.

"Dr. Hoffer and I found the longer the patient is sick, the slower and less certain the recovery," cautioned the delightfully humorous, modest Scottish voice. "But since nothing else has helped and the treatment is harmless, why not try it?"

Circumstances at that time carried me to the East and I consulted with other pioneering doctors in the field: Carl Pfeiffer in Princeton, David Hawkins and Jose Anibal Yaryura-Tobias at the North Nassau Mental Health Center, Manhasset, Long Island, and Allan Cott in New York City.

The night before returning to California, I was introduced to a young woman, Mary, who had recently recovered from schizophrenia herself through nutrition and vitamin therapy. I was so impressed I persuaded Robert's family to hire her to aid in his treatment.

Dr. Pfeiffer agreed to examine blood samples from my patient for histamine, zinc, copper, B_{12}, and folic acid and advised a vitamin and mineral regime. Robert was also placed on a hypoglycemic high protein, limited carbohydrate diet, without refined starches or sugar, and was withdrawn from coffee and cigarettes. Mary, the recovered patient assistant, moved in with the family for a month, instructing them in the diet and starting Robert on a daily physical exercise program.

Passing my Board examinations in Psychiatry in December 1970, I left Robert on his therapeutic regime in Mary's care and embarked with my wife on a long journey around the world.

While in the highlands of New Guinea, we met a Methodist missionary. When the missionary discovered I was a psychiatrist, she invited us back to her mission, saying "I've got a patient for you." Located in a primitive stone-age area, the mission was only forty minutes by air from Mt. Hagen; but the mile-and-a-half jeep ride from the airstrip was two hours on the crude native-built road.

The following day I met Parume, a thirty-five-year-old woman so bedraggled and emaciated she looked fifty. Wearing Campbell's soup cans as arm bracelets and bearing a bag of garbage on her back, Parume greeted me with an appealing but silly smile and laughed bizarrely.

"She has ben sick five years," the missionary said. "Her

husband will not allow her to dig in the family yam patch; her tribe has thrown her out. She would have starved but for us."

Wishing an interview, I requested an interpreter and the mission lady and I retired inside. Suddenly we heard a loud thud, followed by shrieks and moaning from the porch. We rushed out to find Parume lying prone, blood trickling from a gash on her scalp. A couple of frightened native boys had stoned her, such was the terror the mad woman held for her tribe. Parume wasn't seriously injured, and when the interpreter arrived the interview commenced. She felt a divine calling to return the natives to their ancestral Satan worship and away from the colonizers' Christianity. Parume spoke darkly of the skeletons of dead men lying in the jungle and believed she communicated with their spirits. Satan's demons had thoroughly infested her with tormenting aches and pains in her belly and joints. She was indeed what Western doctors would call a paranoid schizophrenic.

What could I do for this madwoman whom I saw for one hour and would never see again? No talk therapy or social work could possibly help because of the insurmountable language and cultural barriers. Only a chemical therapy could work; why not try the megavitamins? "I will give you foods which will slowly drive the demons out of you," I announced in my best witchdoctor fashion. She was pleased and grateful, and the missionary and I retreated inside. We wrote Dr. Pfeiffer, asking him to send niacin, vitamin C, and a B-complex which, along with a high protein diet, was my prescription. The native diet of yams is poor in protein, rich in carbohydrate, and contains a mild hallucinogen, the worst diet for most schizophrenics. The missionaries donated tins of fish, the only available protein.

Five months later, my wife and I returned to California. When I checked on Robert, I found a miraculous transformation.

"Hello, Dr. Lesser. I'm glad to see you," he greeted me in a shy, gentle voice. I was amazed. Before when I had tried to engage him, he would shuffle off to a corner of the room, scratch his head, and gaze vacantly, lost in a private world. Now he was calm and no longer hallucinating or irrational. He watched TV, read for the first time, and kept himself groomed and bathed. Robert no longer wished to run away, but if he had he was no longer so bizarre that he would be picked up by the police. This cure could not be attributed to psychotherapy. I hadn't even been around when his sanity returned. True, Mary had lived with the family for a month and had been immensely helpful in educating them about the diet and in getting Robert off cigarettes and coffee. But schizophrenics had received milieu therapy and social work counseling before without such productive results. The wealthy few lived for years in fine lodgings with highly intelligent, loving, professional social workers and counselors ministering to their every need. These benefits appeared to make little difference in the ultimate outcome of their disease. I felt Robert's recovery had to have been induced by the nutrients and special diet.

A letter arrived from the New Guinea missionaries, bringing a second pleasant surprise. Parume had recovered completely and had been accepted back by her husband and tribe. A few months later, the missionaries sent a second letter. My patient had relapsed. When the missionary investigated, she found Parume's husband had been taking the tinned fish for himself. Restored to her high protein diet, Parume promptly recovered again.

Working on Myself

These two cases stimulated my study of nutrient therapy. Before I started to practice, we spent the summer of 1971 in Big Sur, California, studying the deep tissue massage method, Structural Integration, with Dr. Ida Rolf.[10] After thirty years of sitting at desks and poring over books, like many "educated" people, I'd become alienated from my body. Dr. Rolf's method restores the lithe flexibility we all enjoy as small children.

Structural Integration, "rolfing," requires ten hours of deep, painful massage—painful because muscles held immobile for years, locked in spasm, are suddenly freed by the rolfer's hands.

After the first two hours, I could breathe about twice as deeply as before. My entire body, supercharged with extra oxygen, felt loose and alive. Scurrying down to an ocean cove, I scampered over the rocks like a monkey, delighting in the newfound physical freedom. As the sessions progressed, I did not always leave exhilarated. Sometimes depressed or angry, I felt like running and hiding away. What really hurt was not the physical pain, though the pain involved in unsticking glued-down muscles is often severe, but rather the *emotional* pain some of the sessions unleashed.

Dr. Rolf's technique builds on Wilhelm Reich's theory of character armor. Reich believed strong emotion lodged in the body, causing a rigidity which constricted the tissues and cut off the flow of streaming energy. Rolfing, by loosening the body's soft tissues, unwraps the traumatized, tightened body and exorcises the original negative feelings which froze the body into its rigid immobility, its character armor.

Suddenly two new dimensions, the physical and the chemical, were added to my knowledge of human nature. Their addition gave me a much clearer perspective than I'd had when I had considered only the psychological and social dimensions.

Evolving My Own Form of Treatment

We settled in Berkeley in August, 1971. Harry and Theda Shifs of the San Francisco chapter of the American Schizophrenia Association helped me get started in practice.

The American Schizophrenia Association is a grass-roots organization seeking effective treatment for schizophrenia. It has fifty-six chapters throughout Canada and the United States. The American Schizophrenia Association is a division of the Huxley Institute of Biosocial Research. The Huxley Institute seeks effective treatment not only for schizophrenia, but for all types of mental illness. It provides information, sponsors training, and stimulates research in nutrition and vitamin therapy.

In 1972, I joined the Academy of Orthomolecular Psychiatry, formed the previous year in London. Thanks to these organizations, I was not alone as I struggled to develop an orthomolecular nutritional approach in treating mental illness.

No one prescription of nutrients worked in every case; the vitamins had to be tailored to each individual's needs. Roger Williams, the American chemist who discovered the B vitamin pantothenic acid, showed there are vast differences betwen individuals in their biochemical requirements. I abandoned the search for a universal cure-all and instead sought methods of diagnosing each patient's unique biochemistry.

Some hypoglycemics, for example, did not respond to a

high protein, limited carbohydrate diet. A few only felt well and mentally clear when they ate nothing. These patients seemed allergic to food. Whenever they ate, they became mentally dull, disoriented, confused, and depressed. Their food allergy affected their mind; they had a *cerebral allergy*. Mental imbalance due to an allergic reaction of the brain is often accompanied by physical signs. Cerebral allergy sufferers are "mouth breathers" because their nasal passages are swollen and clogged. There are dark blue shadows under their eyes. The tongue is coated and "boggy"; the face is puffy, the complexion pasty white. These signs can all indicate a chronic food allergy. These food allergy patients were inevitably addicted to their allergy-inducing foods.

I saw several hyperactive children with learning disabilities. They were living on junk foods: refined sugar and salt-laden cereals, chemically saturated ice cream, soda pop, candy, and refined-flour pastries.

To help hyperactive children on junk food diets, I insisted that junk food be kept out of the house. The entire family converted to a diet of meats, fish, fowl, fresh fruits, and vegetables. In addition, I prescribed large doses of vitamin C and the B vitamins niacinamide, pyridoxine, and pantothenic acid. More than half of these children lost their hyperactivity within one month and their performance at school steadily improved.

Politics: A New Idea Encounters Resistance

A new idea always encounters resistance, and nutrition and vitamin medicine is no exception. In July, 1973, the American Psychiatric Association, in *Task Force Report #7*, condemned megavitamin therapy and orthomolecular psychiatry. The politically motivated report fell like a hammer on the infant Academy of Orthomolecular Psychiatry. At the 1973 Academy meeting, held before the issuance of the *Task Force Report*, over 300 attended. In 1974, after the report, attendance dropped to 100.

In early 1975, State Senator James Mills, speaker of the California Senate, announced he would introduce legislation to "further and support orthomolecular psychiatry." A planning meeting was held in San Diego. We wrote one bill to modify Medical, the state health insurance for the indigent, to include vitamins and minerals if prescribed by a physician.

Currently, most drugs prescribed by a physician are covered by Medical. But if the physician wishes to treat his patient's disease with a nutrient, the welfare patient has to find the money to buy it. A second bill required insurance companies doing business in California to provide coverage for orthomolecular medicine. That afternoon, February 15, 1975, we met again and formed the California Orthomolecular Medical Society. I was elected its first president. Starting with ten charter members, the society has grown to a national organization of 400 physicians as of this writing.

The bills passed the California legislature by overwhelming margins, despite opposition from the American Psychiatric Association. But the governor vetoed them.

We reintroduced the legislation the following year (1976), this time limiting the coverage to three counties. Again the legislation passed overwhelmingly; even the American Psychiatric Association offered only token resistance. This time the governor approved and orthomolecular medicine had received its first official sanction and support.

In December, I became a half-time physician at Napa State Hospital. My purpose was to establish an Orthomolecular Ward, where volunteer mental patients could receive nutritional treatment. Seven months later, I was still waiting to begin. The Health Department Committee for the Protection of Human Subjects would not approve the project. They listed so many objections the Director finally ended the program and I left Napa State.

But the patients and parents of patients refused to let nutritional treatment die. A demonstration on the hospital grounds was held and the parents held a sit-in at the state capital. It now looks as if an Orthomolecular Ward will be established after all, though the Committee for the Protection of Human Subjects is still balking.

On June 22, 1977, I testified with other witnesses before the Select Committee on Nutrition and Human Needs of the United States Senate on the subject of nutrition and mental health.[11] This was the fifth in a series of hearings on diet related to killer diseases. Present was Chairman Senator George McGovern and Senators Charles Percy, Robert Dole, and Richard Schweiker. A transcript of the hearings along with a collection of papers on orthomolecular psychiatry was published as *Diet Related to Killer Diseases, V* and is available from Parker House, 2340 Parker Street, Berkeley, California 94704, for $6.95.

Slowly, gradually, nutrition and vitamin therapy is making progress. Organized medicine is beginning to investigate the nutritional approach. Medical students are asking for courses in nutrition. Legislation similar to that passed in California is being prepared in other states. The public and physicians are now seeking greater understanding of the use of nutrients in medicine.

This book presents my experience over the past ten years. We begin in the next chapter with the B-complex vitamins. Following chapters will consider the other vitamins and minerals, and deal with special problems.

The B-Complex Vitamin Family

A vitamin is an organic food substance which occurs naturally only in living organisms. Vitamins are present in foods only in minute quantities, but are absolutely essential for proper growth, health, and life. Fifteen vitamins have been recognized and analyzed, and perhaps others remain waiting to be discovered. Therefore, a truly complete vitamin formula doesn't yet exist. But by using a concentrated natural food, such as dessicated liver or brewer's yeast, to provide any unknown food factors, one approaches a "complete" formula.

Vitamins are of two types: fat soluble and water soluble. Fat-soluble vitamins dissolve in alcohol and are more easily stored in the body. The fat-soluble vitamins are A, D, E, and K. Since water-soluble vitamins dissolve in water, they are much more easily lost by the body through the normal eliminative processes. The water-soluble vitamins include the B series, vitamin C, and the bioflavinoids (vitamin P).

The B vitamins are a "family" because they are found together in the same foods and do similar work in the body. Further, the symptoms of one B vitamin deficiency may be indistinguishable from those of another.

B vitamin deficiencies are very common in our modern diet as the B vitamins (along with vitamin C) are largely lost in food refining, processing, and cooking. Therefore, a B-complex multivitamin supplement is often helpful. If fatigued, tense, or depressed, try a B vitamin complex before a tranquilizer, because the B vitamins are especially important in our energy and nervous functions. As the B vitamins are water soluble, excesses pass out in the urine, making it very difficult to receive an overdose.

Be careful to obtain a B-complex which has adequate amounts of *all* the B vitamins. Many B-complexes are poorly balanced because the manufacturer uses ample quantities of the cheap B vitamins such as niacin but skimps on the expensive ones such as pyridoxine (B_6). Using a balanced B-complex which contains equal amounts of all the B's therefore assures an adequate supply. For common tension or fatigue, I usually recommend a balanced B-50 or B-100, which contains, respectively, 50 and 100 mg of each of the B vitamins.

Brewer's yeast, dessicated liver, and wheat germ are excellent food supplements for obtaining B vitamins in the balanced form existing in nature.

Keeping in mind that for common stress I recommend a balanced combination of all the B vitamins as most sensible, let us now examine the B vitamins one by one, with some true case histories illustrating their specific use.

Vitamin B_1 (Thiamine)

At a state institution I was asked to see Frank, just transferred from prison. He'd been depressed since an evening two years previously when he announced to his girlfriend that it was all over between them. "Stoned" on pot and liquor, the distraught girl grabbed a nearby pistol and blew out her brains while Frank stared, glassy-eyed.

Shaken by her violent suicide, he heard her voice calling to him constantly. He couldn't sleep, ate poorly, lost weight, and harbored suicidal thoughts. Frank had taken antidepressant drugs for over a year with no improvement. Outside, he'd used drugs and alcohol copiously; in the institution, the only stimulant available was strong coffee which he swilled continuously.

Poor diet and caffeine addiction in combination can create a thiamine deficiency, causing depression; I prescribed 500 mg of thiamine twice daily for my new patient. The next day, Frank remarked he'd got his first good night's sleep in two years, and that his depression was lifting. The following day, capitalizing on the looser security of the institution, he escaped and hasn't been seen since. Ironically, the escape can be seen as a sign of improvement, since it required more activity than Frank could have mustered when depressed.

The connection between thiamine deficiency and depression became apparent to me while I was in Manhattan, eating in restaurants, drinking strong New York coffee, and smoking big cigars.

At a luncheon meeting with a husband and wife writing team from a prominent nutrition magazine, the following conversation ensued:

"Hey Doc, I see you're hitting the coffee pretty hard," said the husband.

"Yeah," chimed in the wife, "don't you know coffee can cause a thiamine deficiency?"

A lightbulb switched on in my brain. I *had* been feeling depressed, and I'd also noticed a pins and needles sensation whenever I landed hard on my feet. Immediately after lunch, I gulped down a B-complex containing 50 mg of thiamine. The next day my feeling of well-being returned; and continuing on 50 mg of B_1 daily, within a week I found that the pins and needles, which I'd attributed to old age, had completely disappeared! Of course, I also cut down considerably on coffee.

Recognizing Thiamine (B_1) Deficiency

Mild thiamine deficiency appears as apathy, confusion, emotional instability, irritability, depression, a feeling of impending doom, fatigue, insomnia, headaches, indigestion, diarrhea occasionally but usually constipation, poor appetite, weight loss, and feelings of numbness or burning in the hands and feet (paresthesia).

Anyone thinking thiamine deficiency isn't common may consider the following study[1]: volunteers received the amount of thiamine present in a typical American diet of bread, beef, corn flakes, potatoes, polished rice, sugar, skim milk, canned fruits and vegetables, gelatin, egg white, cocoa, and coffee. To ensure the diet was sufficient in all other nutrients except B_1, it was supplemented with brewer's yeast in which the B_1 had been destroyed by heating. They also received iron, calcium, phosphorus, vitamin C, and halibut liver oil (for A and D), a diet superior to that eaten by millions of Americans.

Within three months, "All the volunteers became irritable, depressed, quarrelsome, uncooperative and, without knowing why, fearful that some misfortune awaited them. Two became agitated, felt that life was no longer worth living and threatened suicide. All became inefficient in their work. In part this could be attributed to weakness, in part to inability to concentrate, confusion of thoughts, and uncertainty of memory. . . ."

Many other complaints were voiced, such as headache, backache, unusually painful menstrual periods, sleeplessness, tenseness, formication (the sensation of insects crawling over the skin), inability to tolerate pain, and sensitivity to noises.

In time, they developed low blood pressure, anemia, and a lowered metabolic rate. Soon they experienced heart palpitations and shortness of breath, developing abnormal electrocardiograms, and in several the heart became enlarged.

When I was a boy, our family doctor advised me to give up athletics because a chest x-ray showed my heart to be enlarged. Now I believe I was suffering from an unrecognized thiamine deficiency, as my diet was similar to that of these Mayo volunteers. Although my physician was conscientious, he never once mentioned vitamins or nutrition in relation to my case. I'm sure it never occurred to him to do so.

The Mayo volunteers' ability to work as measured on an exercise machine decreased as the diet continued, and all their symptoms were made worse by exercise or cold weather. Numbness and pains developed in their legs and feet, and they had little or no hydrochloric acid in their stomachs.

By the twenty-first week, they had such severe headaches, nausea, and vomiting that the experiment was ended. Thiamine (B_1) was added to their supplement without their knowledge to avoid any placebo effect. No other change was made in their diet. Wtihin a few days they became cheerful, lost their fatigue, and reported a feeling of well-being and mental alertness, associated with marked stamina and enterprise. The flow of stomach acid became normal in twelve days, their hearts in fifteen days.

If you suspect thiamine deficiency, your physician can obtain a test for transketolase activity, a measure of blood thiamine. The level of thiamine in the urine can also be measured. As these tests can cost fifty dollars each, it's safe simply to take thiamine for a few weeks.

White rice, white flour, white sugar, and alcohol all contribute to thiamine deficiency by providing calories for your body's machinery, but without the thiamine, stripped in processing, needed to convert these calories into energy. Stimulants like tobacco and caffeine also burn up thiamine, creating deficiency—"nicotine fits" and "coffee nerves"—and all cola drinks contain caffeine, as does chocolate.

Raw fish, clams, and oysters also contain an enzyme (thiaminase) which destroys thiamine.

Stress increases your B_1 need, especially the stress of exercise, so joggers, beware! If exercise, rather than being invigorating, only magnifies your exhaustion, think of thiamine shortage, as B_1 is a necessary cog in the body's energy machine.

How to Get B_1

Rich natural thiamine sources are wheat germ, rice polish, brewer's yeast, and bran. Your body requires 0.5 mg of B_1 for every thousand calories of food.

A 10- to 50-mg capsule daily is ample as a supplement, but since a single B vitamin deficiency rarely exists alone, it's more sensible to take a total balanced B-complex.

Whenever possible, capsules containing the pure vitamin powder are preferable to tablets. Tablets usually contain excipients and binders to hold them together. Some people react badly to these excipients, and the tablets can be compressed so tightly by the tablet-making machines that the vitamins are not completely digested and absorbed.

To treat severe deficiency such as occurs in beriberi, heart disease, or alcoholic polyneuritis, physicians occasionally prescribe much larger doses, 500 mg of B_1 twice daily. Where digestive disturbance puts absorption through the gut in doubt, as in chronic alcoholism, B_1 is given by injection into the muscle.

Vitamin B_2 (Riboflavin)

The depressed widow's eyesight was failing. She was developing cataracts, a clouding of the lens, which would soon need surgical removal. Because vitamin A and riboflavin (B$_2$) are intimately involved with the eye, I placed her on 10,000 IU of natural vitamin A from fish liver oil and 400 mg of riboflavin daily.

No improvement occurred for several months, though her sight ceased to deteriorate. Recently her eyesight has improved and the cataracts are receding.

The potential medical benefit of nutritional therapy is immense. But it requires perseverance. Nutrients *often* require several months to effect a response. But for the patient who *is* patient and sticks to it, real improvement is frequently the reward.

Persons taking a B-complex containing riboflavin often become concerned because their urine becomes bright golden yellow. Riboflavin is bright yellow in color and gives urine this harmless fluorescence.

Recognizing Riboflavin Deficiency

Riboflavin deficiency is only rarely responsible for mental symptoms, though many consider it the most common vitamin shortage in America. Reportedly, a B$_2$ deficiency can cause trembling, dizziness, insomnia, and mental sluggishness. The common symptoms of riboflavin deficiency are a magenta or purplish tongue, cracks in the corner of the mouth, and lips which look chapped. In a long-standing deficiency, the upper lip becomes progressively smaller and practically disappears.

As the shortage becomes severe, the eyes may water and the lids crust and burn. The victim frequently rubs or wipes the eyes. The eyes become bloodshot, and tiny blood vessels appear on the surface of the skin (acne rosacea), most noticeably in alcoholics. The skin becomes oily, with scaling around the nose, mouth, forehead, and ears. Tiny fatty deposits like whiteheads appear.

As sensitivity to noise is an early symptom of thiamine deficiency, sensitivity to light is an early symptom of riboflavin deficiency. Persons who only feel comfortable wearing dark glasses might suspect B$_2$ need. B$_2$ deficiency can cause hair loss, disappearance of the eyebrows, even baldness.

Riboflavin need increases with increasing consumption of protein or carbohydrate. It promotes new cell growth, as in pregnancy, lactation, wound healing, and malignant tumors.

On the other hand, a deficiency of riboflavin greatly increases the cancer-causing potential of some carcinogens.

Sources of Riboflavin

Vegetarians, in particular, are prone to riboflavin deficiency, as animal protein such as milk, liver, tongue, and organ meats are the best natural sources. Brewer's yeast is the richest source.

A 10-mg tablet daily is a quite adequate supplement, unless you are ingesting massive amounts of the other B vitamins, especially B_6, in which case B_2 should be increased proportionately.

Niacin (Nicotinic Acid, Nicotinamide, Niacinamide)

Niacin is often dramatically effective in reversing sensory dysperceptions such as hallucinations, delusional thinking, and disturbances of mood and energy.

Severe niacin deficiency (pellagra) displays the "four D's" of diarrhea, dermatitis (inflammation of the skin), dementia (madness), and, ultimately, death.

By 1914 pellagra afflicted more than 200,000 Americans. No one knew what caused pellagra, and many researchers considered it a contagious infectious illness. Dr. Joseph Goldberger[2] of the U.S. Public Health Service began an extensive investigation of the Southern mental hospitals and orphanages where the disease was rife. He concluded that pellagra wasn't contagious because in every institution where the inmates were seriously ill, the staff members were rarely stricken.

In a Mississippi orphanage, Dr. Goldberger found that nearly half the children had varying degrees of pellagra. Their standard fare consisted of biscuits, hominy grits, syrup, corn mush, and salt pork. He was able to enrich this diet in one ward, adding fresh meat, milk, eggs, beans, and peas. Within a few months, the enriched diet ward was pellagra-free, while the occurrence of pellagra in the other wards remained unchanged.

Continuing his research in a prison, Dr. Goldberger promised eleven inmates freedom in exchange for their living on the suspected diet of biscuits, mush, grits, syrup, coffee, corn, bread, cabbage, sweet potatoes, and rice. In six months, five of the eleven had pellagra.

In 1915, Dr. Goldberger announced his findings that malnutrition was the sole cause of pellagra and proper diet its cure. But some scientists still believed pellagra was a contagious disease.

In 1916, Dr. Goldberger, his wife Mary, and several staff members ingested and injected themselves with the blood, urine, feces, and skin lesion material of pellagra patients, in what they called "filth parties"—a final demonstration that no infectious agents were involved. Of course, no one contracted pellagra; but complete proof that pellagra was due to malnutrition did not come until 1937.

That year nicotinic acid (niacin) was isolated from liver extract and, when fed to a pellagrous dog, produced a rapid recovery. A final puzzle remained. Infants thrived on milk which theoretically seemed deficient in niacin. In 1945 the puzzle was solved when the amino acid tryptophan was discovered. Tryptophan converts to form niacin in the body, and milk is a rich source of tryptophan.

In areas of the world where corn is a basic staple, such as southern India, pellagra still accounts for 8 to 10% of mental hospital admissions.

Identifying Niacin Deficiency

The first noticeable symptoms of niacin deficiency are entirely psychological. Victims may feel fearful, apprehensive, suspicious, and worry excessively with a gloomy, downcast, angry, and depressed outlook. They may experience headaches, insomnia, loss of strength, and burning sensations all over the body. Their depression may range from "blue Mondays" to the wish to end it all. "When the going gets tough, the tough get going," but niacin-deficient people just fold up under stress. They may become alienated recluses, who maintain a marginal existence by determinedly avoiding the stress of life.

In some cases a niacin deficiency may act to dull the moral sensibilities, adversely affecting the individual's behavior. Whereas in most people niacin deficiency causes depression or inability to concentrate, in others it may be the underlying cause of thoughtless promiscuity, pathological lying, or petty thievery. The following is a good example.

Ted's difficulties were the final expression of father-son pathology. Prior to "surrendering his career to the liquor bottle," Dad had been a pillar in the community, president of the Lions Club. After alcohol, he was fit only for president of the Liars Club, maintaining two mistresses simultaneously, unbeknownst to each other, or to Mom. Dad even tried robbery, brandishing a toy pistol in a drunken, bumbling manner, portending the comic-opera style of Ted's life of crime. Because of his standing in the community, charges were dropped.

Ted was a chubby teenager, tipping the scales at 260 pounds. He sought help from the family doctor, who discovered an underactive thyroid. Ted lost twenty pounds on thyroid and water pills before stopping the hormone because it made him nervous. He drifted back to 260 by the time he reached eighteen, whereupon he visited another physician. Again he was prescribed thyroid, along with amphetamine "diet" pills. Ted lost sixty-five pounds and his sanity as well, as the diet pills made his fantasies seem real. Enjoying their effect, he took three times the recommended dose. The pills made him feel he was a "big man"; he used bad checks and credit cards to impress his friends with rented Cadillacs, fancy hotels, and gambling in Reno; completely captured by his fantasies until he was captured by the law.

Ted was twenty-five when I first saw him, newly married and in more legal trouble. His wife was pregnant and he was charged with fraud. Posing as an auto leasing agent, he had collected deposits and never delivered the cars. Free on bail, Ted purchased hefty life insurance policies, making his bride the beneficiary. Telling her his nonexistent "new employer" wanted to give them a honeymoon in Tahiti, he financed the trip with a credit card sent to him by mistake. On the honeymoon he repeatedly tried suicide in ways which would appear "accidental," so his spouse could collect on the insurance policies. As inept at suicide as he'd been at fraud, he was found out by his wife who persuaded him to return to California. Bail jumping was then added to Ted's other legal problems.

For the past six months, anxious about his criminal charges, Ted had been hearing voices and sleeping only four fitful hours nightly.

Psychological testing ordered by the court confirmed Ted to be borderline psychotic, with impaired capacity to discern right from wrong. His nervous remorse and lengthy depression argued against his being a true criminal psychopath, without conscience, as did his genuine concern for his wife and parents. His naive haphazard illegal activities were more in line with the behavior of a disorganized psychotic than that of a cunning psychopath. The amphetamine diet pills, used in excess, had probably driven him over the edge, as amphetamine abuse can precipitate psychosis.

His thyroid tested normal, but the glucose tolerance test I ordered revealed he was hypoglycemic. I placed Ted on a high protein, frequent-feeding diet, without white sugar or refined starches, and a general vitamin plan with 1500 mg of vitamin C and 1500 mg of niacin. Later, zinc and 300 mg of B_6 were added.

Within a week, he stopped hearing voices, slept more soundly, and lost much of his nervousness. Within a month, his depression completely lifted, and he attributed his improvement to the niacin.

"Before, when I got depressed, I would go on into a fantasy. Since I've been taking the niacin, when something depresses me, I'm able to check myself, and I don't slip into unreality."

Ted was sentenced for his prior offenses and went to prison while his wife gave birth to a son. In prison he experienced remorse, developed a religious passion, became an honor prisoner, and decided to enter the ministry.

More Cases of Niacin Deficiency

One August I was consulted by a young man from Montana named Michael, who told me "I'm scheduled to enter medical school in the fall, but my mind is gone."

Early that spring after breaking off with his girlfriend, he had become depressed, lost his appetite, and couldn't sleep. Thinking it might help, he'd taken MDA (a hallucinogenic "street" drug), but he became worse. His memory impaired and unable to study, he barely finished college. He had been accepted for medical school, however, because of his strong prior record. Michael developed an alienated view of the world and felt "stoned" all the time, though he used no more drugs. He became a ravenous junk food "junkie," consuming five or six sugar doughnuts for breakfast and two or three double-dip ice cream cones for lunch.

By summer, Michael had gained over forty pounds, was sleeping only two hours a night, and was experiencing "crazy" thoughts, so he came to California seeking treatment. He saw a "holistic" physician, who placed him on a "cleansing" fruit fast. Two days later he was much worse: heart racing, extremely anxious, and not sleeping at all. The doctor referred him to me. Stopping the fast, I placed him on a high protein, frequent-feeding diet, as his glucose tolerance test revealed relative hypoglycemia. Because of a high blood copper, he was given zinc, 3 g of vitamin C, and rapidly built up to 6 g of niacin for his mental symptoms.

Within three days, he felt immensely better. He lost his "stoned" feeling and was able to sleep. Most importantly, his concentration returned, allowing him to begin medical school a few weeks later. He called recently to say he's starting his third year of school, maintaining his diet, taking 3 g of niacin daily, and feeling fine.

In another case, an unwilling young woman was brought by her worried parents into my office. Believing I was the devil, she would not cooperate. She'd experienced a nervous breakdown five years earlier after her husband of three months had walked out on her. Her condition became chronic; she heard voices, suffered paranoid delusions, and stayed out of the hospital only because her parents tolerated her bizarre behavior. She'd been seeing a psychiatrist three times a week for two years, receiving psychotherapy and tranquilizers which slightly helped her chronic insomnia but hadn't touched her psychosis.

Pork chops, ham, and bacon were the main meats in her diet, and she swilled coffee, sodas, and beer.

I ordered laboratory tests, but fearing the blood drawing would "kill" her, she raced out of the office. Working with her parents, I put her on 1.5 g of niacin, 1.5 g of vitamin C, 200 mg of B_6, balancing multivitamins and a high protein diet, without pork, coffee, sugar, or alcohol.

Six visits and six months later, she was feeling well enough to move out on her own and hold down a full-time job. She gradually lost her fear and became able to form relationships, meeting a young man whom she eventually married. From time to time, she would neglect to take her niacin, fall off her diet, or start drinking beer, any of which precipitated her metabolic madness. Returning to her regime invariably restored her mental health.

The tranquilizer was gradually withdrawn over the first six months, and today, five years later, she requires none, remaining healthy on nutrients alone.

In yet another case, a fearful, bedraggled young woman

came into my office, gloomy and depressed. It was difficult to piece together her story, as her narrative was given in a scattered, disconnected fashion.

She'd had a string of one-night stands, but her mental disorganization prevented her from maintaining a relationship. Unable to concentrate, she hadn't worked in three years, surviving on state aid. Periodically during our interview she burst into tears for no discernible reason.

In a few visits, on 2 g of niacin daily, with a balanced formula of other nutrients and a high protein diet, she became clear-thinking, rational, and dry-eyed. On subsequent visits, I could always tell when she wasn't taking her niacin, as she would again start crying without apparent cause. Once she realized the niacin was helping her, she stayed on her vitamins and got off welfare.

High Protein Diet Makes Niacin Effective

In cases such as these, though niacin was probably the significant factor, the patient is always given the niacin with a nourishing diet and other vitamins and minerals. As Dr. William Kaufman informed me, "You have to take the niacinamide with a high protein diet, or else it is ineffective." Dr. Kaufman has found that 250 mg of niacinamide six times daily, with a high protein diet, brings marked improvement in the treatment of arthritis. He did not give other vitamins, as the patients didn't seem to need them. "The niacinamide appears to make the other vitamins present in the diet more effective."

Niacin, with a diet adequate in protein, is frequently helpful in treating people with severe mental illness. When such persons are on tranquilizers, the dosage can be lowered and sometimes stopped completely.

Physical Signs of Niacin Deficiency

In mild niacin deficiency, the tip of the tongue is usually reddened from engorgement with blood, and the taste buds on the tongue's surface are enlarged, giving a stippled appearance, the characteristic "strawberry tip." Farther back, the tongue is coated white with bacterial growth and debris, often imparting a foul mouth odor. As the deficiency becomes chronic, deep midline cracks and crevices appear. Later, the tongue becomes red and swollen all over, accompanied by dental indentations of the margins, lending it a scalloped appearance. Finally, the enlarged taste buds atrophy, with loss of substance, and the tongue's surface develops a glossy, bald appearance. The mouth becomes sore, the gums swollen and painful.

Digestive disturbances are also present in early niacin deficiency. The stomach secretes little or no hydrochloric acid, absorption of nutrients is impaired, and the person has excessive gas and poorly formed, foul-smelling stools. Since food cannot be digested efficiently when a niacin deficiency has been present, recovery can be slow. Yogurt in copious quantities is helpful at first, because it supplies predigested protein, along with acidophilus bacteria to restore the normal gut flora, which make niacin and other B vitamins for us.

In more severe niacin deficiency, dermatitis (inflammation of the skin) develops symmetrically on exposed areas. First becoming slightly reddened, the skin itches and burns intensely, then becomes tense and swollen and eventually atrophies, its color fading to brown. Darkening of the skin, often seen in the elderly, is possibly partially due to niacin deficiency.

A nationwide survey conducted in 1971–72 by the U.S. Department of Health, Education and Welfare[3] revealed that many Americans had clinical signs of niacin deficiency. The elderly suffered most; 13.2% of those sixty and over had fissures of the tongue. Women from eighteen to forty-four proved slightly more deficient than men of the same age. In addition, 9.2% of women compared with 8.6% of men *above* the poverty level showed serrations and swelling of the tongue, while only 6.2% of the men and 6.8% of the women *below* the poverty level displayed the same clinical signs, suggesting that a higher income doesn't ensure a better diet.

Many more Americans probably suffer from mild niacin deficiency which causes mental fatigue, irritability, weakness, abdominal pains, constipation, or sleeplessness. One reason for widespread niacin deficiency is the American reliance on highly refined, high carbohydrate foods. Niacin, like most B vitamins, metabolizes carbohydrates, so the large amounts of sugars and starches in many processed foods rob niacin needed for other functions. Further, niacin, as other B vitamins, sometimes occurs in bound forms, meaning it is not released from the food to be available to the body. Cereal grains and corn, for example, actually contain considerable niacin, but in an unavailable bound form.

Using Niacin Therapeutically

In using niacin, I begin with a modest dose of 50 mg three times a day and build up to the optimal level, the dose which achieves maximum improvement. Some physicians advise patients to increase their niacin intake to the level at which they first experience stomach upset or diarrhea, and then maintain their dosage 1 g (1000 mg) below this level. I prefer to double the dose every few days until maximum mental improvement has been achieved, generally finding 3 g a day sufficient. Occasionally much larger doses are required. Some patients ingest up to 40 g daily for years with no apparent ill effects, though many will experience nausea, vomiting, diarrhea, or a flu-like syndrome while taking anywhere from 1 to 6 g of niacin a day. When used in larger doses, the vitamin works more like a drug in that it suppresses symptoms; often in such cases some other problem is being missed.

Niacin, like other nutrients, should be taken with meals, as vitamins work together with the food. Further, because niacin is a weak acid (nicotinic acid), it is less likely to upset the stomach if taken with food.

The Niacin Flush

Because niacin releases histamine, a powerful dilator of the surface blood vessels, doses of 100 mg or more often cause a warm flush of the skin, making it tingle and giving it a reddened, sunburned look. This flush generally occurs within fifteen to thirty minutes after niacin ingestion, though on occasion it may appear as much as two or three hours later; and some never experience the flush at all. If niacin is used continuously, the flush becomes less pronounced, but if it is discontinued a few days and then reinstated, the flush will again be strong. The flush is an "all or none" reaction and does not become more severe if the dose is increased.

The skin flush and the patient's reaction to it often indicate whether niacin will be helpful. Those who don't need niacin will complain bitterly about the flush. Those whom niacin helps don't mind the flush, or tolerate it because of the dramatic clearing of perception and increased energy they experience. Some even enjoy the "rush" or "high" of the flush. Those so disoriented they are literally "outside their skins" find the flush puts them in touch with their bodies.

Whenever considering niacin to treat severe mental illness, the physician should test the patient's *blood histamine* level; this test indicates how well an individual will respond to niacin. Persons high in histamine (histadelic), about 20% of the population, flush strongly from niacin, and some even experience headache (histamine headache). Such people usually don't benefit from niacin. Those low or normal in histamine experience a less severe flush and are likely to be helped by niacin. The histamine test is expensive, costing about $60, but a rough measure of histamine can be obtained through an *absolute basophil count* for only about $5. The higher the basophil count, the higher the histamine level. A basophil count of 0 or 1 indicates low or normal histamine, while 2 or more basophils means high histamine.

The heavier the meal taken with the niacin, the less severe the flush. Cold liquids suppress the flush, while hot liquids or hot baths make it more pronounced. Taking an antihistamine (Periactin, 4 mg) fifteen minutes before taking niacin will suppress the histamine reaction and suppress the flush.

Niacinamide (*A Flushless Form of Niacin*)

Niacinamide (nicotinamide), the amide of niacin, does not cause the skin flush and provides a useful alternative when the flush is not considered desirable, as in the treatment of children. But in the treatment of alcoholics, the amide is ineffective whereas niacin reportedly is often effective in reducing the craving for alcohol and increasing the patient's feeling of well-being. Further, niacinamide does not lower blood cholesterol, while niacin does; and in depressed adults niacinamide may be more toxic than niacin. One woman, who had been taking 26 g of niacinamide daily for several months when I first saw her, had nausea, indigestion, an enlarged liver, and swelling of both legs. Discontinuing the niacinamide resulted in prompt clearing of her symptoms. A young man developed patches of increased skin pigmentation (*acanthosis nigricans*) on 3 g daily of niacinamide; these faded a few weeks after he stopped taking it.

Conditions Where Niacin Should Be Avoided

Persons taking medication for high blood pressure cannot at the same time take niacin safely, as a full dose may cause a marked drop in blood pressure.

Nicotinic acid should also be avoided in active ulcer disease, because of niacin's acidity. But if the ulcer sufferer needs niacin, potassium nicotinate is reportedly tolerated well.

Because niacin raises the uric acid level, it may bring on an attack in those suffering from gout. And since niacin raises blood sugar, diabetics may need to increase their insulin. For the same reason, hypoglycemics (low blood sugar) are often helped with niacin.

Though it is not known whether niacin can be toxic to the liver, persons with active liver disease should avoid large doses.

Other Uses of Niacin

Dr. Edwin Boyle found that in a group of 160 heart patients taking 3 to 4 g of niacin daily over a ten-year period, the actual death rate was only 10% of that expected. Niacin improves blood circulation, thus its favorable effect on the heart. For the same reason, niacin may help in the treatment of intermittent claudication, poor circulation of the extremities. This also possibly explains its benefit in treating Ménière's syndrome (vertigo) and in lowering cholesterol and reducing high blood pressure. Niacin has also been reported helpful in aborting migraine attacks, increasing stomach acid in impaired digestion, and treating acne.

Getting Enough Niacin

The recommended daily allowance is 18 mg for men, 13 mg for women, and 9 to 16 mg for children, but the optimal dose varies widely from individual to individual and increases markedly with stress.

Lean meats (not pork), poultry, fish, and peanuts are rich sources of niacin, as are the dietary supplements brewer's yeast, wheat germ, and dessicated liver.

Vitamin B$_6$ (Pyridoxine)

Sandra, a plump woman with a pale blond complexion, visited from Oregon. She was worried she would lose her accounting job because she fell asleep on her feet for a few minutes every three or four hours, often causing her to make embarrassing mistakes. Sandra's sudden sleep attacks were symptoms of narcolepsy, an epilepticlike condition of unknown cause. During these attacks, her heart would pound and jump into her throat, her neck seemed to swell to twice its size, and she felt she was leaving her body and floating in the air. Her attacks were more likely to occur when she was frightened and under stress.

Present since youth, the condition was becoming more severe as she grew older. Lately she had experienced abdominal pains, fatigue, sluggishness, and severe emotional ups and downs. Often she felt she was "going crazy."

During a six-hour blood sugar test, administered by another physician, her back, which had pained her in the past, began to ache after the third hour. Soon she was dripping with perspiration, felt faint, and lost consciousness before the physician gave her an injection (probably sugar water) which revived her. Sandra's blood sugar at that point of unconsciousness was a very low 30 mg% (30 mg of blood sugar in 100 cc of blood), confirming the presence of hypoglycemia (low blood sugar). For several days following the test, she felt unwell. The doctor placed her on a frequent-feeding hypoglycemia diet and, discovering she was anemic, gave her iron.

Though the diet helped Sandra, the frequent eating caused her to gain weight. When she came to me she weighed 155, up from her ideal 118 pounds. Fat as a child, Sandra managed to stay slim only by strict dieting, which the hypoglycemia no longer allowed. Like many hypoglycemics, she had no appetite in the morning, but once she started eating she became ravenous.

She was a divorcee and blamed herself for not having remarried: "A number of good men have been interested, but as soon as they get to know me they don't call anymore." Nearing forty, she despaired of ever finding a lasting relationship.

"Are you having any other problems?" I inquired.

"I feel depressed most of the time, especially before my periods, which have never been regular," she said, smiling. "I have very severe menstrual cramps and suffer terribly. If I didn't have strong religious convictions," she added, increasing her smile, "I believe I would end it all."

Smiling depression is not uncommon; many depressives maintain a brave front, but Sandra's performance went beyond the common. She exhibited what psychiatrists call "la belle indifférence"; she described her most sad and desperate situation in a bland, unconcerned manner, as if it were happening to someone else. Only her suicidal ruminations revealed that Sandra was all too painfully aware of her suffering.

"Do you dream at night?" I asked.

"I can't remember the last time I had a dream," she replied.

"And do you have stretch marks on your skin?" I continued.

"Yes, around my hips and stomach, and here on my upper arms; but I suppose that's because I'm fat."

Dr. Carl C. Pfeiffer of the Brain Bio Center, Princeton,[4] has described a certain type of mental illness the victims of which are blonde, blue-eyed, and have a sallow complexion. Like Sandra, they have stretch marks on their hips and thighs, are nauseous in the morning, and don't dream or don't remember their dreams. They may have neurologic symptoms, like Sandra's narcolepsy, and women have irregular menstrual periods. They have an iron-resistant anemia which responds to B_6 and show white spots on the fingernails, probably a sign of zinc deficiency. I examined Sandra's fingernails; they were riddled with white spots.

In addition to my usual testing, I ordered a urine analysis for kryptopyrole, the mauve factor, as Pfeiffer's work showed that kryptopyrole is elevated in this syndrome. For elevated kryptopyrole, Dr. Pfeiffer prescribes vitamin B_6 and zinc, which lowers the kryptopyrole to normal and concurrently helps the mental illness.

"Right after you have your lab tests," I told Sandra, "I'd like you to take six drops daily of this zinc solution and 100 mg of B_6 twice a day with meals. Look for dreaming," I instructed. "If after three nights you don't dream, and remember the dream in the morning, then double the B_6 to 200 mg twice daily. If after three nights at the higher dose you still don't dream, phone for further directions."

Large doses of pyridoxine will stimulate dreaming in anyone. Persons who habitually do not dream, or cannot remember their dreams, are able to dream normally with sufficient B_6 and zinc.

Sandra telephoned a week later. "I had one fleeting

dream the first night I increased the pyridoxine to 400 mg a day, but none since," she reported. "Still, I have more energy and feel better!"

"Double the B_6 again to 800 mg daily; we've got to get you to dream. When you have dreams and are able to remember them in the morning, we'll know you're receiving enough pyridoxine. Double those zinc drops from six to twelve, and take 800 mg of B_1 and B_2 and four tablets of chelated magnesium, because all these work with the B_6," I explained. "Come see me in a week, and we'll go over your lab tests and see how you're doing."

Sandra bounced into my office a week later and happily announced her daytime sleeping episodes had completely disappeared. She had begun dreaming and could recall her dreams in the morning. She began to describe one of her dreams when I interrupted her. "Hold on, right now I'm only interested that you *are* dreaming."

Many of the white spots on her fingernails were gone, and no new ones were forming. Her lab tests still indicated mild anemia, though she'd been taking iron for months, and her kryptopyrole was abnormally high. Increasing her pyridoxine to 1000 mg a day, I asked her to return in three weeks.

At our next appointment, a man accompanied her to the waiting room. In the office, she beamingly reported further good news. She had experienced her first painless period ever, her depression had lifted, and her mind was functioning more clearly. She was developing a trim figure, finding it easy to lose weight. The man in the waiting room was her boyfriend, and they were already talking about marriage.

"I think this is the last time I'll be seeing you, Doctor," she announced. "I'm cured!"

Congratulating her, I cautioned her to check with me again in three months.

That was five years ago; her urine kryptopyrole became normal, her anemia cleared, her depression and narcolepsy disappeared, she kept her accounting position—plus she married the guy. Sandra maintains her health on 400 mg of vitamin B_6 a day, plus other balancing nutrients.

Detecting B_6 Deficiency

Pyridoxine (B_6) deficiency is perhaps the most common vitamin deficiency cause of epilepticlike nervous symptoms and hysterical, explosive, labile, "emotionally upset" depression. Sufferers are painfully shy, sick recluses who must avoid other people, though they maintain a good intellectual grasp and are free from delusions and hallucinations.

As in Sandra's case, an iron-resistant mild anemia is present in B_6 deficiency. The red blood cells are smaller in size and deviate in shape from their usual uniform circular disclike form.

Low blood sugar is common in B_6 deficiency, causing headache, dizziness, irritability, inability to concentrate, and extreme weakness. Excessive body weight, much of which is often retained water, is shed quickly when B_6 is provided. People deficient in B_6 may have dandruff in "showers" on the shoulders and oily scales on the scalp and eyebrows, around the nose, and behind the ears. Sufferers may experience numbness and cramping in the arms and legs. Their hands may be dry, cracked, and ache painfully, while mouth and tongue are also cracked and sore. Nausea, especially in the morning, and insomnia are other prominent symptoms of pyridoxine deficiency.

Theraputic Uses of Pyrodoxine

Vitamin B_6 in doses of 75 to 1000 mg per day, along with magnesium and other nutrients, is helpful in treating many childhood disorders, loosely classified as *autism*.[5]

Convulsions in infants, "rum fits," and other epileptic-type illnesses sometimes respond to pyridoxine. It can help certain cases of Parkinson's disease, the morning sickness characteristic of pregnancy, adolescent acne, and some anemias which do not respond to iron.

Ten milligrams of B_6 and three hundred milligrams of magnesium oxide completely prevent the recurrence of kidney stones in 79% and benefited 89% of 265 patients with long histories of recurrent stone formation.[6]

Pyridoxine need is increased by estrogen, the female sex hormone, and pyridoxine supplements are helpful in situations where elevated estrogen levels exist. Serious deficiencies of B_6 are reported[7] in 50% of women taking birth control pills and experiencing mood changes, such as pessimism, irritability, tiredness, depression, and loss of sex drive. In a group of such women given 20 mg tablets of pyridoxine hydrochloride twice daily for two months, those women who were B_6 deficient experienced relief from the symptoms of depression. Many women became depressed and tense before the onset of their menstrual cycle, and these *premenstrual blues* can often be eliminated by 50 to 200 mg of B_6 daily. Pregnancy also increases estrogen levels and consequently seems to increase pyridoxine requirements.[8]

A diet high in sugar (sucrose) or in protein, especially the amino acid methionine, increases B_6 need, as do the drugs isonicotinic acid (an antituberculosis medicine), hydralazine (for high blood pressure), and certain antibiotics. On the other hand, the B vitamins pantotheninc acid, choline, biotin, and the essential fatty acids all have a pyridoxine-sparing effect, decreasing the need for B_6. B_6 supplements decrease the toxicity of the insecticide Dipterex, barbiturates, carbon monoxide gas, and x-rays.[9]

Getting Enough B_6

The recommended daily allowance of pyridoxine is 2 mg per day, but when it is used to treat symptoms, anywhere from 5 to 1000 mg daily may be required. Anyone taking more than 50 mg of B_6 a day should take balancing amounts of the other nutrients used in pyridoxine metabolism. A magnesium deficiency may be created by large doses of B_6 without supplemental magnesium; therefore, I prescribe four tablets of chelated magnesium (2000 mg of magnesium amino acid chelate, equivalent to 400 mg of elemental magnesium) daily. Riboflavin and Thiamine are also desirable in doses equal to the amount of B_6 employed, and zinc (80 mg of zinc sulfate daily) is particularly important. Brewer's yeast, two heaping tablespoons daily, is a necessary general supplement for optimal B_6 metabolism.

Food Sources

Meats, especially organ meats, fish, whole wheat bread, soybeans, avocados, peanuts and walnuts, fresh fruits, particularly bananas, and vegetables are all good natural providers of B_6; wheat germ is the richest source. These foods are also good sources of the other nutrients used with B_6, revealing the perfect balance present in nature. Raw sugar cane, for example, contains goodly amounts of B_6, helpful in metabolizing the sugar, but this B_6 is refined out in the preparation of white sugar.

Pantothenic Acid (Calcium Pantothenate)

The most prominent mental symptom of the B vitamin pantothenic acid deficiency is fatigue, but insomnia, sullenness, and depression can also occur. Calcium pantothenate deficiency may be realted to the nervous disease and psychosis seen in some alcoholics (Korsakoff's Psychosis).[10]

The "Antistress" Vitamin

Pantothenic acid can be thought of as the antistress vitamin, helping with stress-induced fatigue because of its effect on the adrenals, our "antistress glands." A deficiency of pantothenic acid causes adrenal exhaustion, and eventual destruction of the adrenal glands. Humans suffering fatigue related to adrenal exhaustion may experience an ache in the small of the back, where the adrenal glands are located. If you are fatigued or suffering from allergies because of stress, and a good night's sleep doesn't correct the problem, try 250 mg of calcium pantothenic a day. If you suffer one cold after another, consider pantothenic acid, as frequent respiratory illness can signify a deficiency. Pantothenic acid with B_6 and folic acid is necessary to manufacture disease-fighting antibodies.

Does your mate complain that you grind your teeth in your sleep, and suggest separate bedrooms? Before you move out, try pantothenic acid with some calcium. Dr. Emmanual Cheraskin[11] successfully treated a series of sixteen tooth grinders (tooth grinding is called bruxism) with nutrients, the most vital of which appeared to be pantothenic acid and calcium. Probably these particular vitamins helped because tooth grinding is thought to be a sign of unconscious stress. Calcium helps because a lack of calcium will cause muscles tenseness and cramps. The powerful jaw muscles are a prime spot for stress-induced tension to lodge.

Volunteers at Iowa State Prison were given a diet adequate except in pantothenic acid.[12] They became fatigued after two weeks of deprivation, lost their appetites and were constipated by the third week, and became quarrelsome, belligerent, and discontented by the fourth week. Adrenal hormones measured in the urine fell progressively lower as the experiment continued. The volunteers also developed low blood pressure, stomach distress, and continuous respiratory infections, with reduction in stomach acid and enzymes. By the fifth week, the volunteers were quite miserable and burning feet added to their suffering. At that point it was necessary to end the experiment. All symptoms disappeared when pantothenic acid was returned to the diet.

Getting Enough Pantothenic Acid

Roger Williams, the discoverer of pantothenic acid, recommends 250 mg twice daily to treat any stress-induced symptons.[13] Brewer's yeast is the richest natural source, followed by organ meats, bran, peanuts, and peas. A natural diet assures sufficient pantothenic acid, as it is present in nearly all foods; the vitamin's name is derived from *pantos*, the Greek word for everywhere. Eating excessive processed foods, however, may create a shortage, as much is lost in refining (e.g., 50% in the milling of flour).

Vitamin B_{12} (Cobalamin)

Vitamin B_{12}, nearly always given by injection, is helpful in two kinds of mental illness, one rare, the other common.

Pernicious Anemia

The rare mental illness is associated with pernicious anemia, called pernicious because if not corrected it is fatal. When B_{12} is lacking, the bone marrow (the body's blood cell factory) is unable to produce healthy red blood cells. A long-standing deficiency of cobalamin (B_{12}) causes neurologic degeneration with numbness, tingling, unsteady gait, loss of reflexes, etc.

Three to five years before the anemia or neurologic changes occur, however, almost any type of mental symptom may appear: apathy, mood swings, poor memory, disturbances in concentration and learning, auditory hallucinations, confusion, paranoia, and psychosis.

B_{12} Shots for Fatigue

The common mental condition for which B_{12} injections are employed is tiredness and nervousness of a general sort, unrelated to the rare pernicious anemia. Family physicians have used B_{12} shots for years in treating these conditions, despite criticism by colleagues that the shots have only a placebo effect. Doubting doctors may read "A Pilot Study of

B_{12} in the Treatment of Tiredness," by Ellis and Nasser,[14] where under double-blind conditions, hydroxycobalamin (B_{12}) injections were demonstrated to be decidedly superior to injections of a placebo.

B_{12} shots often rescue old people labeled as having senile psychosis. H. Wiek et al.[15] found B_{12} deficiency in 58% of 138 such cases of psychosis and organic brain syndrome, and Dr. Carl Pfeiffer[16] states that "schizophrenia" first appearing in the middle age or old age is usually due to a B_{12} deficiency.

Vitamin B_{12} sometimes stimulates growth in malnourished, undersized children. It also plays a part in maintaining fertility and stimulating the production of breast milk.

The Tongue in B_{12} Deficiency

In B_{12} deficiency the tongue becomes strawberry red, as in niacin deficiency; but whereas niacin deficiency increases the bud "bumps" at the tip (strawberry tip), with cracks and a white debris coating further back, in B_{12} deficiency the tongue is smooth at the tip and sides and shiny red all the way back.

Getting Enough B_{12} (Food Sources)

Dietary lack as a cause of B_{12} deficiency is rare, but as we receive B_{12} almost exclusively from animal products (meat, poultry, fish, eggs, brewer's yeast, and dairy products), deficiency does occur in strict vegetarians. Nutritionists have observed that though some British vegetarians have developed pernicious anemia, the disease is rare among Indian vegetarians. Probably this is because Indian vegetarians eat yogurt which contains B_{12}.

B_{12} is stored in the liver, which in a good nutritional state contains 2 to 5 mg, enough to last three to five years.

Supplements

The usual dose of hydroxycobalamin for treating mental symptoms is 1000 micrograms once or twice weekly, injected subcutaneously. The hydroxycobalamin form is superior to cyanocobalamin because it maintains an active bloodstream level longer. B_{12} is available in tablets for oral administration without a prescription, but since susceptible persons lack an intrinsic factor in the stomach cells which permits B_{12} to be absorbed, it is more effective when taken by injection.

Folic Acid (Folacin, Folate)

Folic acid and B_{12} are intertwined biochemically, and folic acid deficiency also produces an anemia. Cracks and scaling on the lips and at the corners of the mouth (cheilosis), usually identified with a riboflavin deficiency, can also indicate folate deficiency.[17]

Folic acid deficiency is much more common than B_{12} deficiency. Though I routinely measure both B_{12} and folic acid in all my patients, I have only occasionally found a low B_{12} level, but low folate levels are present in nearly 20%. Folic acid is the most common vitamin deficiency I have documented.

Mental Symptoms of Deficiency

As in B_{12} deficiency, long before an anemia develops, mental symptoms of folate deficiency appear.[18, 19] Poor memory is particularly prominent, possibly because folic acid is needed in the synthesis of nucleic acids such as RNA (ribonucleic acid), which appears important in the storage of recent memory events. Apathy, withdrawal, irritability, and slowing of the intellectual processes are the other mental symptoms associated with folic acid deficiency.

Deficiency is particularly likely in the elderly; one study of elderly persons unable to care for themselves found 67% folate deficient. As with B_{12}, folic acid deficiency creates a vicious cycle by preventing the stomach from producing digestive acid and destroying the small intestine's mucosal lining. This causes a malabsorption syndrome, further aggravating the nutrient deficiencies. One wonders how many senile nursing home residents, where the average life expectancy from day of admission is six months, are suffering from folic acid deficiency. At least partial reversal of such senility sometimes occurs through good nutrition with nutrient supplements, including 1 mg of folic acid twice daily and weekly B_{12} shots.

Epileptics on anticonvulsant medication such as Dilantin and Myselin may experience folic acid deficiency because these drugs destroy folic acid. These antiepileptic medications cause apathy and slowing of mental processes, probably

because of the induced folate deficiency. Giving epileptics
folic acid improves their drive, mood, intellectual speed, alertness, concentration, self-confidence, independence, and socia-
bility, but folate deficiency in epileptics should be corrected
cautiously, as doing so occasionally increases the frequency
and severity of their fits.[20]

As with thiamine, alcoholics are very likely to be deficient in folic acid because of the intestinal malabsorption
caused by drinking.

Because folic acid corrects the anemia of B_{12} deficiency,
thereby masking the need for cobalamin (B_{12}), and since
folate cannot reverse or prevent further neurologic damage
resulting from B_{12} lack, the government has banned the sale
of folic acid supplements stronger than 0.4 mg without a
doctor's prescription. Obtaining a blood count and a B_{12}
level before treating folic acid deficiency guards against this
rare hazard.

Getting Enough Folic Acid

One milligram of folic acid twice daily with meals for
two to three months is sufficient to correct a deficiency and
replenish the liver stores. A well-stocked liver will provide
adequate folate for seven to nine months, giving the person
time to increase the consumption of leafy green vegetables.

As with B_6, increases in estrogen lower folic acid levels,
so women taking birth control pills and pregnant women
should probably take a supplement.

Foliage, liver, and yeast are the richest natural sources
of the vitamin. Folic acid was first identified in spinach, and
the name folic is taken from *folium*, the Latin word for leaf.

Choline

A young woman burst into my office, arms flailing about
uncontrollably as she lurched into a chair. Her guttural
speech was barely distinguishable because her mouth was
grimacing repeatedly, completely out of her control. Every
few seconds her tongue would dart out of her drooling
mouth, serpentlike.

Mentally disturbed since infancy, she had been on tranquilizers for ten years. Her writhings and contortions were
the unfortunate effects of these phenothiazine tranquilizers.

This condition, termed tardive dyskinesia, develops in 30 to 45% of patients taking phenothiazine-type tranquilizers for an extended period of time. Once it develops, the condition is permanent, with no known cure. Recently, however, it was discovered that 10 to 60 g daily of the B vitamin choline improved 50 to 75% of tardive dyskinesia cases.[21]

Part of the B-complex, choline is the essential component for acetylcholine, a substance which transmits nervous impulses across the gaps between nerves in the nervous system. Increasing the activity of acetylcholine may be the mechanism by which choline corrects tardive dyskinesia.

I was not able to use choline in this case, because the girl suffered from epileptic seizures and large doses of choline may worsen eiplepsy.

Tragic cases such as this make me cautious about prescribing tranquilizers and strengthen my conviction that nutritional therapy is the correct path. The physician's responsibility, said Hippocraties, is "First, do not harm."

Drugs are chemicals foreign to the body which can easily be abused and cause harm. Nutrients, even if taken in excess, are relatively safe. No one has ever committed suicide with an overdose of a vitamin. What drug has such an enviable record?

Choline is also helpful in treating cirrhosis, the "fatty liver" alcoholics and others on high-fat, low-choline diets develop. In a group of 158 patients with hypertension, choline dropped the blood pressure of all within three weeks, the pressure of one-third of the patients falling to normal.[22]

Getting Enough Choline

Choline is a constituent of lecithin. A heaping tablespoon of granular lecithin contains 500 mg of choline, which helps lower blood cholesterol by aiding in its removal from the bloodstream and its use in metabolism.

Other rich dietary sources are egg yolk, brewer's yeast, fish, soybeans, peanuts, beef liver, and wheat germ.

Inositol

"I sleep fitfully, half-awake, until around noon," my patient groaned, "wake up feeling drugged and half-dead until about sunset, and don't begin to feel decent until late evening. I like to stay up at night, because it's quiet, and my mind becomes active. Actually, it's too active; by eleven o'clock when I should sleep, I feel incredibly alive and my brain is jumping! I take a tranquilizer and a sleeping pill to fall asleep . . . usually I need two or three. So how can I function, Doc, and work, when I can't even get to sleep?"

I nodded sympathetically, recalling sleep-deprivation studies which showed that even the healthiest subjects hallucinate and become psychotic if deprived of sleep too long.

"I don't like using tranquilizers and sleeping pills to get to sleep. They leave me feeling drugged the next day, and I wake up hardly rested."

I nodded again, aware that sleeping pills do not provide the same quality of sleep as when it's naturally induced. Recent studies indicate sleeping pills can actually cause insomnia if used habitually over a period of time. Further, not a few insomniacs, in desperation to get a "good night's sleep," have taken overdoses of sleeping pills, never to wake up again.

"There is a nutrient which may provide nighttime sedation," I responded. "It's inositol, a B vitamin. Get some 500-mg tablets at the health food store and take one to three at bedtime. It's quite safe at that level; actually, as much as 50 g (50,000 mg) has been taken by mouth with no ill effect."

The next week my patient reported, "That inositol is subtle, but it did calm me so I was able to sleep better. It's not like a sleeping pill . . . it didn't knock me out, but I felt mellow and didn't get so excited I couldn't sleep."

If the inositol hadn't been successful—and often it isn't —I'd have suggested megadoses of vitamin C, chelated magnesium, or the amino acid L-tryptophan, other nutrients which provide sedation and aid sleep. Large doses of these nutrients may be required before they make you sleepy, and they don't always work at any dose. But they generally don't cause a hangover, aren't habit-forming, and the desperate patient who takes an overdose won't wind up in the county morgue.

Inositol has a mild anti-anxiety effect, similar to the effect of mild tranquilizers such as Valium or Equanil. Sometimes it is a useful alternative; Valium can't lower cholesterol or blood pressure, or help remove fatty deposits in the liver, but inositol can.

Getting Enough Inositol

Though present in very high quantities throughout the body, especially the brain, inositol's metabolic function is obscure. It is also unknown how much inositol is needed, or if it's needed at all, since apparently it can be synthesized in the body. Inositol is richly present naturally in lecithin, beef brain and heart, wheat germ, bulgar wheat, brown rice, brewer's yeast, molasses, nuts, and citrus.

Biotin

Though no psychiatric benefit from supplements of the B vitamin biotin has been found, it is used successfully to treat certain common skin inflammations in infants.

Biotin deficiency has been produced in humans in two different ways: consumption of many raw egg whites (about 30% of the total diet) for an extended period of time, and use of too many antibiotics, which destroy biotin-producing intestinal bacteria. Raw egg white contains avidin, a carbohydrate-containing protein which binds biotin, preventing its absorption. Cooking the egg white inactivates the avidin, allowing biotin, unharmed by heat, to be absorbed. Raw egg lovers be warned!

Sydenstricker[23] fed four volunteers a diet deficient in biotin. Within five weeks they developed a flaking, itchless inflammation of the skin, with a grayish pallor, mental symptoms of depression, drowsiness and lassitude, nausea and loss of appetite, muscle pains, and heightened sensitivity to touch. Later, anemia, elevation of blood cholesterol, and changes in the electrocardiogram occurred.

Food Sources

The average diet provides ample biotin; rich sources in addition to egg yolk are organ meats, yeast, legumes, and nuts.

PABA (Para-aminobenzoic acid)

PABA is a little-known member of the B-complex family, unique in that it is a vitamin within a vitamin, forming a component of folic acid.

Problem schizophrenics have been given 2 g of PABA a day with reported good results.

Dr. Ana Aslan, at her longevity clinic in Rumania, advocates procaine injections (H_3 or Gerovital, an acidified form of procaine buffered with potassium) to retard aging and even to reverse some of its effects. Procaine (novocain) is the local anesthetic commonly used by dentists, and PABA makes up part of the procaine molecule. When procaine is broken down in the body, PABA is released.

PABA is of further interest because of its rumored ability to reverse graying of hair. Pantothenic acid, biotin, folid acid, and vitamin E also enjoy a similar reputation, though no studies have demonstrated conclusively that any of these vitamins can reverse gray hair.

PABA is used to treat Peyronie's disease, an affliction of men past middle age in which the tissue of the penis becomes abnormally fibrous, causing a marked curvature of the phallus on erection, which is usually painful. PABA's helpfulness in this condition is based on its apparent ability to increase oxygen supply to tissues. In twenty-one patients placed on PABA for periods ranging from three months to two years, pain on erection disappeared in all sixteen cases where it had been present, and the penile deformity objectively improved in ten of seventeen patients. The average dose is 12 g, usually given as four 500-mg tablets six times a day. At these levels, loss of appetite, nausea, and skin rash occasionally occur.

Rich natural sources of PABA are liver, yeast, wheat germ, molasses, and eggs. PABA also serves as an excellent sun screen when applied to the skin, and various ointments are available for that purpose.

Pangamic Acid ("Vitamin B_{15}")

In 1951, E. T. Krebs isolated pangamic acid from apricot pits and assigned it the fifteenth place in the vitamin B series. In the strict sense, however, "B_{15}" isn't a vitamin at all, because it has not been proved an essential dietary requirement the absence of which would lead to deficiency or disease. Despite its ambiguous nutritional status, pangamic acid has been widely studied[24] and accepted in many countries (primarily the Soviet Union) as a necessary food factor with important physiological actions.

Dr. Allan Cott, a nutrition-oriented psychiatrist, believes B_{15} benefits about 25% of the disturbed children he sees, primarily by stimulating speech in children whose speaking ability is retarded. Dr. Bernard Rimland, director of the Institute for Child Behavior Research in San Diego, believes "B_{15} makes autistic kids more normal. It helps correct a wide range of behavior disturbance." He feels that pangamic acid has anti-allergenic properties, and that diseases like autism may be allergies of the nervous system.

The Russians have studied B_{15} most intensively and report it useful in treating alcoholism and other drug addictions, autism, schizophrenia, minimal brain damage, senility, aging, heart disease, diabetes, hypertension, liver disease, poisoning, and skin disease—in short, just about anything.

A food substance which can treat "just about anything" has aroused the ire of the Food and Drug Administration, which has seized several shipments of Aangamik 15, the brand name for the calcium salt of B_{15}, which is still available in health food stores ($8.00 per hundred 50-mg tablets), pending the outcome of a court trial.

Meanwhile, many aging athletes chomp down B_{15} like candy. Soviet experiments on swimming rats and human rowers showed it decreased the buildup of lactic acid, the cause of muscle fatigue. Dick Gregory, the comedian and civil rights crusader, takes B_{15} before running marathon races.

The Russians, administering 50-mg tablets of B_{15} twice daily to chronic alcoholics for twenty to thirty days, found in the majority of cases that the alcoholics lost their craving for alcohol. American researchers treating autism and learning disorders in children gave them 50 to 100 mg three times daily and reported no side effects at these levels. Pangamic acid appears to be quite nontoxic; the lethal dose for a 150-pound human is estimated to be 2.2 pounds.

Weakness, fatigue, stomach upset, skin rashes, depression, and ultimately madness and death are the results of B vitamin deficiencies. A healthy gut is essential, both to provide good absorption of the vitamins and to support the normal intestinal bacteria that manufacture many of the B vitamins. An unprocessed natural diet of fresh vegetables, whole grains, and meats will protect most people from B vitamin shortage. Some, however, may require massive B vitamin supplements to fight disease, and most would probably function better and enjoy more optimal health using a regular B vitamin supplement.

TABLE 1

THE B-COMPLEX VITAMIN FAMILY
Use Only Under a Physician's Guidance

B VITAMIN	SYMPTOMS AND SIGNS OF DEFICIENCY	RECOMMENDED DAILY REQUIREMENT	SUPPLEMENTAL DOSAGE	THERAPEUTIC DOSAGE	RICH NATURAL SOURCES
THIAMINE (B_1)	Apathy, confusion, emotional instability, depression, feelings of impending doom, fatigue, insomnia, headaches, indigestion, diarrhea or constipation, poor appetite, weight loss, numbness or burning in the hands or feet (paresthesia), inability to tolerate pain and sensitivity to noises, low blood pressure, anemia, low metabolism, shortness of breath, heart palpitations, enlarged heart on x-ray	0.5 mg per 1000 calories of food	10 mg daily	500 mg twice daily; if malabsorption, given by injection	WHEAT GERM, RICE POLISH, BREWER'S YEAST, BRAN
RIBOFLAVIN (B_2)	Magenta tongue, cracks in lips and corners of the mouth, sensitivity to light, trembling, dizziness, insomnia, mental sluggishness, watery and bloodshot eyes; oily scaly skin with surface blood vessels and whiteheads; hair loss, cataracts	10 mg daily	10 mg daily	Up to 5000 mg daily	MILK, LIVER, TONGUE, ORGAN MEATS, BREWER'S YEAST
NIACIN (NIACINAMIDE)	Fear, apprehension, excessive worry, suspicion, gloom, depression, headaches, insomnia, loss of strength, burning sensations, amoral behavior, sensory dysperception. "Strawberry tip" tongue, red at the tip, coated white with midline cracks and dental indentations at the margins. Foul breath, sore mouth, swollen and painful gums; digestive disturbances, excessive gas and poorly formed foul-smelling stools; dermatitis (skin inflammation); abdominal pain	18 mg—men 13 mg—women 9-16 mg—children	50 mg daily	100 to 10,000 mg	LEAN MEATS, POULTRY, FISH, PEANUTS, BREWER'S YEAST, WHEAT GERM, DESSICATED LIVER

VITAMIN B₆ (PYRIDOXINE)	"Epilepticlike" nervous symptoms; hysteria; "emotionally upset" depression; iron-resistant microcytic anemia; low blood sugar; excessive weight due to water retention; showers of dandruff; oily scaling around scalp, eyebrows, nose and behind ears; numbness and cramping in the arms and legs; cracks on mouth, tongue and hands; morning nausea; insomnia	2 mg	10 mg	100 to 1000 mg	MEATS, esp. ORGAN MEATS, FISH, WHOLE WHEAT BREAD, SOYBEANS, AVOCADOS, PEANUTS, WALNUTS, FRESH FRUITS, esp. BANANAS, WHEAT GERM
PANTOTHENIC ACID (CALCIUM PANTOTHENATE)	Fatigue, insomnia, sullenness, depression, adrenal exhaustion, aching pain in small of back, frequent respiratory illness, loss of appetite, constipation, quarrelsomeness, low blood pressure, burning feet	10 mg	250 mg	500 to 2000 mg	BREWER'S YEAST, ORGAN MEATS, BRAN, PEANUTS, PEAS— present in all natural foods
VITAMIN B₁₂ (COBALAMIN)	Pernicious anemia (megaloblastic, macrocytic); neurologic degeneration, numbness, tingling, unsteady gait, loss of reflexes, mental illness (apathy, mood swings, poor memory, disturbances in concentration and learning, auditory hallucinations, confusion, paranoia, psychoses), shiny red smooth tongue, "tiredness," "nervousness," senile psychosis	6 micrograms (.006 mg)	100 micrograms daily	Hydroxy-cobalamin: 1000 micrograms by subcutaneous injections, once or twice weekly	MEAT, POULTRY, FISH, EGGS, BREWER'S YEAST, DAIRY PRODUCTS
FOLIC ACID (FOLACIN, FOLATE)	Anemia (megaloblastic), poor memory, apathy, withdrawal, irritability, slowing of intellectual processes, cracks and peeling of the lips and corners of the mouth (cheilosis), malabsorption	200 micrograms	0.4 micrograms daily	2 to 40 mg daily	LEAFY GREEN VEGETABLES

B VITAMIN	SYMPTOMS AND SIGNS OF DEFICIENCY	RECOMMENDED DAILY REQUIREMENT	SUPPLEMENTAL DOSAGE	THERAPEUTIC DOSAGE	RICH NATURAL RESOURCES
CHOLINE	Symptoms of deficiency in humans unknown; kidney and liver disorders in rats	Unknown: the amount in a good diet varies between 500 and 900 mg daily	1 tablespoon lecithin	10 to 60 g per day to treat tardive dyskinesia	LECITHIN, EGG YOLK, BREWER'S YEAST, FISH, SOYBEANS, PEANUTS, BEEF LIVER, WHEAT GERM
INOSITOL	Symptoms of deficiency in humans unknown; untreated diabetics lose large quantities in the urine	1 g a day in the diet: it may be made in the body; methionine aids body synthesis	500 mg	3 g daily	LECITHIN, BEEF BRAIN AND HEART, WHEAT GERM, BULGAR WHEAT, BROWN RICE, MOLASSES, BREWER'S YEAST, NUTS, CITRUS
BIOTIN	Flaking, itchless skin inflammation with grayish pallor, depression, drowsiness, lassitude, nausea, loss of appetite, muscle pains, heightened sensitivity to touch, anemia, elevation of blood cholesterol, electrocardiogram changes	Unknown: can be made in man by healthy intestinal bacteria	Unnecessary unless consuming biotin-destroying raw eggs		EGG YOLK, ORGAN MEATS, YEAST, LEGUMES, NUTS
PABA (PARA-AMINOBENZOIC ACID)	Symptoms of deficiency unknown: useful applied to skin as a sunscreen; possible benefit in prolonging life and reversing gray hair	Unknown		12 g's a day to treat Peyronie's disease; 2 g daily for problem schizophrenics	LIVER, YEAST, WHEAT GERM, EGGS MOLASSES, EGGS

The preceding table records B vitamin deficiency symptoms, the recommended daily requirement, the supplemental amount safe to take, and the amount which may be used therapeutically, but only under a physician's guidance. Also included are the richest natural food sources of the vitamin.

4

Vitamin C and the Bioflavinoids

If one could take only a single vitamin, it should be vitamin C (ascorbic acid). Though most living organisms manufacture their own vitamin C, humans and other primates must obtain it from food or die of scurvy. In nearly all mammals vitamin C is produced in the liver from the blood sugar, glucose. But humans, monkeys, guinea pigs, Indian fruit-eating bats, and red-vented bulbul birds lack the enzyme which enables the liver to synthesize ascorbic acid from the closely related common carbohydrate glucose sugar (see Figure 4). Ascorbic acid is produced enzymatically from glucose sugar in all plants and nearly all animals. We also produce ascorbic acid commercially from glucose, usually from corn sugar.

The function of vitamin C in the body is not completely understood. Chemically it acts as a reducing agent; that is, it causes the subtraction of oxygen or the addition of hydrogen in chemical reactions, resulting in the loss of positive charge and the gain of negative charge.

Vitamin C concentrates in the organs and tissues of high metabolic activity: the adrenal and pituitary glands, the brain, eyes, ovaries, and other vital tissues. Any form of stress results in a sudden precipitous drop in the body's vitamin C level. One of the most important functions of ascorbic acid is in the synthesis and maintenance of collagen, the proteinlike "cement" that supports and holds the body's tissues and organs together. Collagen cannot be formed without ascorbic acid, and without collagen, our body's most extensive tissue system, we would disintegrate or dissolve away. When vitamin C is lacking, it is the disturbance in collagen production that causes the fearful aspects of scurvy, the brittle bones that fracture at the slightest impact (collagen provides bones with their elasticity and toughness), the weakened arteries that rupture and bleed, etc. The gradual deterioration of collagen formation is intimately involved with the entire aging process.

FIGURE 4

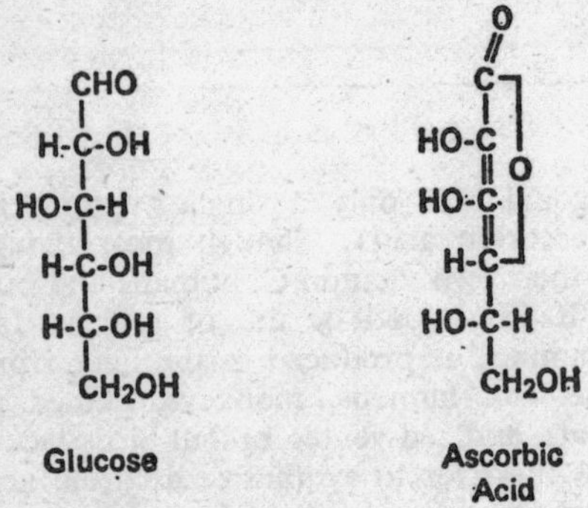

CHO
H-C-OH
HO-C-H
H-C-OH
H-C-OH
CH₂OH

Glucose

O
C
HO-C
HO-C O
H-C
HO-C-H
CH₂OH

Ascorbic
Acid

Vitamin C acts in the body as a potent detoxifier. It negates the effects of heavy metals such as lead, mercury, and arsenic, the carbon monoxide and sulfur dioxide of air pollution, and many carcinogens which, if not detoxified, can cause cancer. Vitamin C increases the therapeutic effect of different drugs and medicines, such as aspirin and insulin, while at the same time reducing their toxic side effects. In large doses, vitamin C has antiseptic and bacteriocidal qualities. In *very* large doses (10 to 1000 g), it even helps kill viruses.

Severe deficiency of vitamin C results in scurvy, the symptoms of which include hemorrhage into the muscles and skin, tenderness and aching of the joints, a general weakening of connective tissue, lethargy, loss of appetite, and anemia. Scurvy's onset is heralded by a failure of strength, the vitamin becoming rapidly exhausted at any effort. The skin becomes sallow or dusky. The gums swell and ulcerate, the teeth drop out, and the breath becomes foul. Blood penetrates the muscles and other tissues, causing severe bruising. In the final stages, profound exhaustion and diarrhea, as well as pulmonary and kidney trouble, lead to death.

Vitamin C and the Mind

Mental symptoms of vitamin C deficiency are fatigue, listlessness, lassitude, confusion, and depression. The face wears a haggard, frowning, "pained" expression, with a careworn, knitted brow.

Confusional states in the elderly, often mistakenly considered senility, may be due to vitamin C deficiency and, if so, will clear with 1 g (1000 mg) daily for three weeks.

Vitamin C in doses of 1 to 2 g at a time works as a tranquilizer for the anxious. Because of the vitamin's sedative effect, similar doses help the insomniac fall asleep.

The influence of vitamin C on the mental state is quite remarkable. Because of the body's homeostatic mechanism, a person can increase his intake of vitamin C 10,000 times over and only double the level of vitamin C in the brain.[1] But that doubling may affect the mental well-being tremendously. Some voyagers in cosmic consciousness claim megadoses of vitamin C are superior to psychedelics, meditation, and EST for achieving a state of bliss. Vitamin C, incidentally, along with niacin, has been used for "coming down" from bad LSD trips.

Fever, overactive thyroid, or stress of any type burns vitamin C excessively, which may explain why 3 to 30 g of vitamin C daily are helpful in severe mental illness, where the sufferer is stressed by extreme anxiety. Possibly vitamin C acts to detoxify a brain poison, as vitamin C helps convert a body chemical, adrenochrome, to leucoadrenochrome, a nontoxic substance. One theory of schizophrenia is that the adrenochrome is instead converted into adrenolutin, a toxin which causes hallucinations and bizarre sensory dysperception.

Megadose C for Schizophrenia and Drug Addiction

Schizophrenics appear to need much more vitamin C than do other people. Vandercamp[2] in 1966 found schizophrenics required doses of 10 to 30 g of vitamin C before they began excreting traces in their urine, indicating they had received enough vitamin C to saturate their tissues. This was ten times as much vitamin C as a control group of normal subjects required.

Megadoses of vitamin C are also useful in treating heroin addiction. Thirty to fifty grams given daily in divided doses by mouth every waking hour provide addicts a smooth, symptom-free withdrawal from the narcotic, reported Drs. Alfred Libby and Irwin Stone.[3]

When such large doses of vitamin C are used in treating drug addiction and schizophrenia, the ascorbic acid form of the vitamin causes hyperacidity in the stomach and swells the belly up like a balloon, because ascorbic acid is a weak acid. I prescribe the sodium and calcium salts of ascorbic acid (sodium ascorbate and calcium ascorbate), because they do not cause hyperacidity when ingested; the acid charge of ascorbic acid is neutralized by the sodium (Na) or calcium (Ca) ion. The sodium or calcium ascorbate forms of vitamin C can also be injected directly into the veins, whereas injecting the ascorbic acid form would damage the tissues.

A very high protein diet is given along with megadose vitamin C to help calm schizophrenics and reduce the withdrawal symptoms of drug addicts. The treatment is effective with tobacco, alcohol, or almost any substance addiction, reports Dr. Libby, provided the addict truly wishes to stop and follows the regime.

Currently, heroin addicts are treated with methadone, a synthetic distant cousin of heroin; treatment consists of substituting a legal addiction for an illegal one. Methadone's only advantages are that it can be taken by mouth and it doesn't provide a "high." If Drs. Stone nad Libby's findings prove conclusive, their nutrient regimen provides a truly superior treatment for heroin addiction.

Methadone is a drug with an infamous history. Spawned in Nazi Germany by I. G. Farben, the giant German chemical complex, it was named Dolaphine in honor of Adolf Hitler. I. G. Farben's industrious chemists also introduced heroin, through their Bayer division. Heroin was originally marketed as a cure for morphine addiction and as a cough suppressant, especially effective in children![4] I. G. Farben also gave the world poison gases, first used by the German military in World War I. I. G. Farben's Zyclon B poison gas was used to murder "inferior" races in the Nazi concentration camps of World War II. Methadone (Dolaphine) was developed as a synthetic substitute for morphine in preparation for that war.

For two years I served as a lieutenant commander in the U. S. Public Health Service at the Federal Correctional Institution, Terminal Island, California. My job was director of a narcotics addiction rehabilitation unit. We never used methadone; we believed you don't cure drug addiction by substituting another drug. Instead, we employed group therapy extensively and developed a "therapeutic community," as first described by Maxwell Jones and John Cummings. We encouraged the incarcerated male and female addicts to face the human problems and pain which had resulted in their seeking an escape into heroin addiction. On the principle of fighting fire with fire, we used ex-addicts as co-therapists to bridge the gap of mistrust.

At the time I knew very little about the therapeutic value of nutrients, but the addicts received nutritious food and performed extensive physical exercise in addition to their regular work. Group meetings were almost continuous. It was amazing to see pale, skinny "junkies" develop into mature, healthy citizens with this therapeutic community approach. The therapeutic community created a "utopian" caring society based on the Golden Rule; it was in everyone's best interests to watch out for and help each other.

Eighty-six percent of the addicts were still out on the street, not fixing, six months after leaving the program.

Addicts tell me that methadone is harder to kick than heroin. I can only hope that high-protein, megadose vitamin C detoxification centers will quickly replace methadone maintenance centers. For those addicts who won't stop, the British plan of supplying legal narcotics through physicians to registered addicts removes the criminal aspects of the problem. When heroin is illegal, addicts may have to steal or get others hooked to pay for their expensive habit.

Vitamin C Raises the I.Q.

In a controlled study of 351 students, those with higher blood vitamin C levels scored an average of 5 points higher than those with lower vitamin C levels. When those with low vitamin C levels were given supplementary orange juice for six months, their I.Qs. (Intelligence Quotient) increased by 3.54 points.[5]

The Optimal Amount of Vitamin C

There is no set amount of vitamin C appropriate for everybody at all times. Need varies from day to day, depending on an individual's amount of stress. The vitamin C requirement may vary from one individual to another by thirty to forty times, perhaps more. One hundred to two hundred milligrams daily, the amount present in a "good" modern diet, is sufficient to saturate the bloodstream.[6] But our ancestors probably received more than 100 mg of vitamin C a day. Nobel Prize-winning chemist Linus Pauling tested the amount of vitamin C present in 110 raw natural plant foods and discovered an average 2500-calorie diet would contain 2300 mg of vitamin C. If the fourteen plants richest in vitamin C were eaten, 2500 calories would provide 9400 mg. From this, Pauling concludes the optimum daily dose of vitamin C lies somewhere between 2.3 and 9.4 g (1 g equals 1000 mg).

But there are other factors even the eighty-year-old Pauling, who takes 10 g of vitamin C a day, doesn't mention. Primitive people didn't breathe smog, drink water through copper pipes (copper inactivates vitamin C), eat food preserved with nitrates (C suppresses the tendency of nitrates to form cancer-causing nitrosamines), or smoke cigarettes (each cancer stick neutralizes 25 mg of vitamin C). Primitive people weren't exposed to x-rays which lower the vitamin C level, or subjected to lead, mercury, and cadmium pollution (vitamin C helps pull these heavy metal poisons out of the body), and life in the prehistoric jungles had to be less stressful than the Manhattan jungle and the Los Angeles tar pits.

Stress greatly increases the need for vitamin C. No wonder Dr. Fred Klenner, who reports he can clear *any* viral illness within 48 hours with enough vitamin C (up to 100 g a day),[7] personally takes 20,000 mg (20 g) daily. Dr. Klenner, still active, is ninety-five.

How much vitamin C should you take? We really don't know. Ten to twenty milligrams daily prevents death from scurvy. One hundred milligrams is present in a typical "good" diet. One reason Pauling and Klenner take such large doses is that animals which can manufacture their own vitamin C produce proportionately high doses. A 150-pound goat, for example, produces 13 g a day. A 150-pound mouse would synthesize 19 g a day, and a rat between 4 and 16 g a day, depending on whether the rat is contented or tormented, illustrating the importance of varying the dose of vitamin C to meet the degree of stress.

Ames Medical Laboratory makes a urine test dip stick (C-stick) which changes color if vitamin C is passing into the urine. If vitamin C appears in the urine, a person can assume his body is getting enough. The C-stick is available through pharmacies.

You can be intuitive about your vitamin C need. If you're having a stressful day, starting to scowl and feeling tense, take vitamin C until your feeling of well-being returns.

More Benefits of Vitamin C

If the smog index is high, your eyes are smarting, and your throat is scratchy from pollution, extra vitamin C offers cellular protection, along with vitamins A and E for the membranes of your lungs. The same goes for tobacco smoke pollution.

I am not perfect; I often smoke cigars while writing. Because of this reckless and nasty habit, my wife and son exile me to my study where I must close all the doors to protect the innocent. As I write and smoke feverishly, the air becomes dense and gray. Gradually my inspiration flags, my thoughts become pessimistic and my writing argumentative. At this point I scurry into the kitchen, tap a gram or two of ascorbic acid powder into a glass, squeeze in the juice of an orange or lemon for the bioflavinoids, swig it down, and return to my typewriter, optimism restored!

Numerous studies have demonstrated that tobacco smoking lowers body vitamin C levels. Pelletier demonstrated that the ascorbic acid (vitamin C) levels of the blood of smokers were only about 40% those of nonsmokers. Two grams daily of vitamin C given to the smokers eventually brought their blood vitamin C levels up to about the same levels as the nonsmokers', though they still excreted less vitamin C in their urine. My advice to smokers is to stop. But if you can't or don't choose to, 2 g of vitamin C daily may provide some protection against the risks of smoking.

Any increase in serum copper increases the need for vitamin C, and estrogen (the female sex hormone) increases serum copper. Therefore, the use of birth control pills (containing estrogen), the use of estrogen medication to prevent menopausal symptoms, and the later stages of pregnancy (when the estrogen level is high) all increase the need for vitamin C. Smoking also increases copper levels, which may explain why vitamin C levels are lowered in smokers. In women, total ascorbic acid (vitamin C) levels are highest at the time of ovulation and lowest at the time of menstruation.

Recall that vitamin C, through its effect on collagen, helps maintain the integrity of bones, cartilage, and connective tissues. Dr. James Greenwood, Jr., professor of neurosurgery at Baylor University College of Medicine, reported in 1964 that vitamin C is helpful in treating lower back pain and its use often prevents the necessity of spinal disc surgery.[8] He recommended the use of 500 mg daily, increasing to 1000 mg per day if there was any discomfort or if strenuous work or exercise was anticipated.

Many have taken up running recently to keep fit, and many are now nursing sore backs. Jogging on hard pavement, especially if the jogger is weighted down with middle-aged spread, is dangerously stressful for spines where the interconnective tissue is depleted of vitamin C. If runners take ample vitamin C, perhaps the spinal discs will be strong enough to endure the pounding stress.

Present in very high concentrations in the adrenal glands, the antistress glands, vitamin C is an important antistress factor, whatever the source of stress—extreme weather, surgery, final exams, or watching the television news.

Spongy, puffy gums which bleed easily, encouraging pyorrhea, signify a possible deficiency. Vitamin C also helps maintain normal vision; cataracts have been produced experimentally by restricting C intake.

Since vitamin C is needed to build new blood cells, anemia can signify a deficiency. Also, vitamin C enhances iron absorption, thereby helping prevent iron deficiency, the most common cause of anemia.

Vitamin C lowers serum cholesterol levels by assisting in the production of hormones from cholesterol and the elimination of excessive cholesterol as bile salts.

Vitamin C may make antibiotics more effective in lower dosages. Workers at the National Cancer Institute have shown that 5 to 10 g of ascorbic acid per day by mouth doubles or triples the rate at which lymphocytes, our body's infection fighters, are produced. Lymphocytes also destroy cancer cells.

The Russians have used it as a muscle builder for their athletes and to retard the aging process.

Most studies indicate daily supplements of 500 to 2000 mg of C reduce the likelihood of contracting the common cold. Linus Pauling's scholarly book *Vitamin C and the Common Cold*[9] discusses these findings in detail.

Vitamin C and Cancer

An elderly Nevada couple entered my office. The patient, was so depressed she could only sit mutely, crying softly to herself, while her husband explained.

"Rosa did O.K. until the menopause. Then she got blackout spells and felt faint and light-headed. She was hospitalized for depression and given tranquilizers and shock treatments, which didn't help. That was twenty years ago. An endocrinologist gave her injections of estrogen which helped somewhat for a while. But these black periods kept coming back. This last episode started a year ago, with back and chest pains. Rosa had a five-hour glucose tolerance test, which dropped sharply in the middle. Her heart was pounding and she had cold sweats. The doctor said she has low blood sugar."

I nodded in agreement, as the relationship between blood sugar abnormalities and depression is well documented, though many physicians remain unaware of the connection.

"She feels worse in the morning," her husband continued. "It's a deep, deep depression. She is agitated and nervous. Last February she tried to kill herself, and the doctor put her on antidepressant drugs. Rosa got better over the summer, but now she's bad again."

The couple hoped there might be a nutritional answer to Rosa's depression, and I ordered my usual biochemical workup. The tests showed Rosa was severely anemic, and the white blood cells (the body's infection fighters) were greatly increased in number. Her B vitamin folic acid level was low, as was her vitamin A level, and her liver tests were elevated, indicating liver impairment. Most disturbing of all, her serum copper was sky high, the highest copper I'd ever seen. High copper can signify an active cancer. Phoning her house, I discovered her medical doctor had already found a malignancy of the blood and she was in the hospital for removal of her spleen, a method of slowing the progress of the cancer.

Three months later, on anticancer drugs, Rosa returned for treatment of the still-present depression. Severe insomnia was a major poblem. I placed her on L-tryptophan, 1.5 g at bedtime to help her sleep, and another 0.5 g in the morning. Tryptophan, an essential amino acid, often helps relieve depression. She also received the B vitamin inositol and chelated magnesium at bedtime to aid sleep. She had a low magnesium level in her hair. As part of her general antidepression nutritional regime, Rosa received 3 g of vitamin C daily. Three weeks later, now well enough to talk for herself, Rosa reported that she was sleeping better and that the depression was lifting. Her medical doctor found that her alkaline phosphate enzyme, high in active blood cancer, had fallen to normal. The vitamin C was doubled to 6 g a day, which decreased the nausea caused by the anticancer drugs. At Rosa's next visit, she announced happily that her depression was completely gone. Her cancer was also remaining in remission, allowing her doctor to reduce her Prednisone, an anti-inflammatory hormone used to fight cancer. Though the medical doctor, pleasantly surprised at the remission in what had seemed a virulent cancer, credited the improvement to the anti-cancer drugs, I wondered if it might have occurred because of the vitamin C (she was now taking 12 g daily).

Linus Pauling, working with Ewan Cameron, a Scottish physician, reported that 10 g of vitamin C daily had increased survival time in 100 terminal cancer patients over four times that of a control group not receiving vitamin C. A fraction of the vitamin C-treated patients were no longer showing any signs of malignancy, though all the control group had died.[10] Although large doses of C seem to help only a minority of terminal cancer patients, perhaps Rosa was one of the lucky responders whose cancer was controlled by her accidental use of vitamin C as part of a general antidepression program.

Precautions About Vitamin C

It has been reported that vitamin C supplements, coupled with calcium, may cause calcium oxalate kidney stones in women. If one takes magnesium as well, that risk is removed. But in a poll I conducted of over one hundred physicians practicing vitamin therapy, no one had ever seen a case where vitamin C caused kidney stones. The rumor appears to be a myth.

A word of caution from Linus Pauling: when one sharply increases vitamin C, the body's enzyme systems, accustomed to a lower intake, shift to accommodate the high C level. If one then abruptly stops the supplemental C, the ascorbic acid in the blood is rapidly converted to other substances by the "revved up" enzymes. The C blood level becomes abnormally low and the resistance to disease may be decreased. This rebound effect lasts for a week or two, until the enzymes decrease to normal for the low vitamin C intake. Accordingly, whenever reverting to a low vitamin C level after maintaining a high intake, decrease the dose gradually over a few weeks.

Vitamin C Toxicity?

Vitamin C appears extremely safe. It has been estimated that one would have to imbibe over *eight pounds* of the powder to reach a lethal dose. Diarrhea would occur long before. Diarrhea appears to be the only unpleasant effect of an overdose of vitamin C. The gut's tolerance of vitamin C increases when illness strikes.[11] This increased bowel tolerance during disease permits larger therapeutic doses by mouth to fight the disease.

Obtaining Vitamin C

Citrus fruits are the most concentrated sources, but leafy green vegetables, tomatoes, berries, and peppers are also rich in vitamin C. One cup of peppers contains 192 mg of vitamin C, one cup of strawberries 88 mg, one cup of parsley 103 mg, one cup of lemon or orange juice 122 mg, and one cup of cauliflower 671 mg. Cooked meats of all types contain only negligible amounts.

Since vitamin C is inactivated in an alkaline medium, adding baking soda to food substantially reduces its vitamn

C content. The vitamin C content of food is preserved by keeping it cool and away from sunlight. Drying and refrigeration help retain vitamin C, while heat and copper inactivate it. Thus cooking foods in copper pans means maximum loss of C. Pickling, salting, curing, fermenting, and leaching all cause nearly complete loss.

Raw cow's milk contains 25 to 30 mg of vitamin C per liter, but pasteurization, by heating the milk, destroys about half of the vitamin C. Human breast milk contains four to six times as much vitamin C as cow's milk. Since there is usually no vitamin C loss before consumption, the occurrence of scurvy in breast-fed infants is negligible. Canned fruit juices, if carefully prepared, retain up to 90% of their vitamin C; but if they are allowed to stand for three or four hours at room temperature exposed to the air, about half of the vitamin C will be lost.

Which is Better, Synthetic or Natural?

There is no such thing as a truly natural vitamin C supplement. The only truly natural vitamin C is that present in foods. On the other hand, there is no such thing as a truly synthetic vitamin C, since "synthetic" vitamin C is created from natural organic chemical sugars. Noted vitamin C authorities Linus Pauling and Irwin Stone feel ascorbic acid ("synthetic" vitamin C) is best, because ascorbic acid is ascorbic acid regardless of its source, and the synthesized form is far cheaper. Since ascorbic acid has the biologic activity of "natural" vitamin C, why not use it? Further, it's easier to take megadoses of the synthetic because it is more easily concentrated. Taking all the extra factors included in natural vitamin C is superfluous and may complicate the biochemical system unnecessarily.

But I am uncertain. I have a lingering suspicion that ascorbic acid might be handled better by the body if presented with the bioflavinoids and other factors with which it appears in the natural state. Paper chromatographs of synthetic ascorbic acid and all-natural rose hip vitamin C present different visual images. The synthetic ascorbic acid looks pale and subdued, almost an outline version of the richer, more lustrous natural vitamin C. Dr. David Hawkins, Director of the Manhasset Mental Health Center, Manhasset, Long Island, says, "There's life energy in the natural rose hip vitamin C, and no life energy in the synthetic ascorbic acid. Kirlian photography reveals a different picture. The natural vitamin C emanates a much more radiant design than the ascorbic acid." Still, this is largely a moot point, as there is precious little natural vitamin C around. Vitamin labels often deceptively tout "All-Natural Vitamin C With Rose Hips" for a product almost entirely synthetic ascorbic acid with a pinch of rose hip powder. Though misleading, this practice is legal, as the Food and Drug Administration considers ascorbic acid to be vitamin C.

How to Take Vitamin C

I use either natural vitamin C or ascorbic acid. I use only powders or chewable tablets which I can convert to powder in my mouth.

When using ascorbic acid powder, mix it in fruit juice, as the acidity of the juice helps preserve the ascorbic acid, and the other constituents of fruit juice, such as calcium and other trace elements, bioflavinoids, and pectin, may enhance the effectiveness of ascorbic acid. Ascorbic acid powder is cheap, available for under $20 per kilogram (1000 g).

I ingest from 1500 to 3000 mg of vitamin C a day in the form of chewable 300-mg tablets derived entirely from oranges. In periods of severe stress I greatly increase my vitamin C intake up to 10 g daily with ascorbic acid powder in orange juice. I generally take one-fourth to one-half teaspoonful of the powder at a time (one teaspoonful equals 4 g of ascorbic acid). Large doses of vitamin C will speed the healing of cuts and burns. When one is stricken with a cold or the flu, large doses (10 to 20 g a day) of vitamin C will suppress the symptoms. Take 2 g every hour to fight a cold or other viral infection. One to four grams of vitamin C will help sober up the intoxicated quickly.

Remember, with vitamin C it's easy to take too little but difficult to take too much. Take vitamin C with meals to prevent diarrhea. If diarrhea occurs anyway, reduce the intake of vitamin C until diarrhea stops. The stomach's tolerance of vitamin C increases if illness is present, reports Dr. Robert Cathcart, III, who has treated 7000 cases with vitamin C.

You can use the sodium ascorbate form to avoid ascorbic acid's acidity, but not if you're on a low sodium diet. In such a case, the calcium ascorbate form is useful.

Vitamin P (Bioflavinoids)

Albert Szent-Györgyi, who received the Nobel Prize for Medicine in 1937 for crystalizing and isolating vitamin C in 1928, also discovered bioflavinoids, brightly colored substances which appear in fruits and vegetables, along with vitamin C. The bioflavinoids are effective in preventing fragility and permeability of the capillaries in guinea pigs. They have been used in medicine to treat dozens of disorders believed related to faulty capillary function, including habitual and threatened abortion, excessive bleeding after delivery (postpartum hemorrhage), nosebleed, skin disorders, diabetic retinitis, bleeding gums, heavy menstrual bleeding, hemorrhoids, and asthma.

Capillaries are the tiny blood vessels which connect the arteries to the veins. Capillaries are permeable, permitting oxygen and other nutrients to flow out into the body's cells, and allowing cellular waste products to flow into the capillaries to be carried off by the veins. If these capillaries become too fragile, they rupture and blood flows into the body's tissues. When this bleeding occurs under the skin, it produces a bruise.

Dr. Thomas Dowd, team physician for the Philadelphia Eagles football team, gave bioflavinoids to the players. After a regimen of three citrus bioflavinoid capsules daily, the number of football players with large bruises after a game decreased from 40% to only 5%.[12]

Dr. Carl Pfeiffer of the Brain Bio Center has given rutin (one of the bioflavinoids) to volunteers in 50-mg doses and measured their brain waves. The results of the quantitative EEG (brain wave test) indicate rutin has both a sedative and a stimulant effect, prompting Dr. Pfeiffer to prescribe 50 mg of rutin every morning for depressed patients.

Clinical studies indicating vitamin P's benefits have not been rigorous enough to convince American scientists, and the therapeutic benefit of the bioflavinoids remains in doubt. The bioflavinoids are reported to act together with vitamin C, prolonging its effects by preventing the destruction of C by oxidation. But Dr. Edme Regnier reported that vitamin C acting alone and vitamin C plus the bioflavinoids were both equally effective in averting the common cold when taken at the first signs of illness (sneezing, scratchiness of the throat, nasal secretion, and chills). Bioflavinoids alone and placebos alone were ineffective.[13]

Others have used the bioflavinoids in treating menstrual disorders (irregular or painful menstrual flow) and find them helpful. The improvement is progressive, the most improvement being reached by the third menstrual cycle.

The bioflavioids are water-soluble; any excess will pass out in the urine. They are nontoxic and without apparent side effects.

Obtaining the Bioflavinoids

The bioflavinoids showing the greatest biological activity are those present in the rind and pulp of citrus fruits. Oranges and lemons are particularly excellent, the pulpy portions of the fruit containing ten times as much bioflavinoid as is found in the strained juice. Frozen orange juice is a relatively poor source of the vitamin P complex because the bioflavinoids give an off taste to the juice, so the amount of pulp squeezed is carefully controlled by the processors. It has not been determined whether humans require bioflavinoids, and therefore no daily requirement has been set.

The richest natural sources are citrus fruits, apricots, cherries, grapes, green peppers, tomatoes, papaya, broccoli, and cantaloupe.

There is abundant evidence that a regular vitamin C supplement will benefit just about everyone. Linus Pauling has concluded that for most people, the improvement in health associated with the ingestion of the optimum amount of ascorbic acid would result in an increase of life expectancy of twelve to eighteen years. In addition, vitamin C shows great clinical promise as a therapeutic agent. Early studies indicate its usefulness in the control of mental illness, viral and bacterial infections, pollution problems, and even some cancers. Governmental and academic medical centers need to study its potential.

The demand for vitamin C by the American public is increasing; we now consume about two pounds of ascorbic acid per person each year.

TABLE 2

VITAMIN C (ASCORBIC ACID)
Use Only Under a Physician's Supervision

SYMPTOMS AND SIGNS OF DEFICIENCY	RECOMMENDED DAILY REQUIREMENT	SUPPLEMENTAL DOSAGE	THERAPEUTIC DOSAGE	RICH NATURAL SOURCES
(Acute scurvy)	20 mg	1000 to 2000 mg daily.	Acute viral illness (colds, flu, etc.) 1 to 2 g every waking hour	CITRUS FRUITS, GREEN VEGETABLES, TOMATOES, BERRIES, PEPPERS, CAULIFLOWER, PARSLEY
Sallow or muddy complexion, loss of vigor, lassitude, tire easily, breathlessness, disinclination for exercise, loss of appetite, anemia, desire for sleep, fleeting pains in joints and limbs, especially legs, bruising		If a smoker, minimum of 2 g (2000 mg) daily	Sudden stress (infection, wound, burn, etc.) 1 to 2 g every waking hour	
(Later stage)			Confusional "senility" .1 to 2 g daily	
Sore gums which bleed readily and are congested and spongy; reddish spots, small hemorrhages on skin, especially the legs at sites of hair follicles; purple and swollen eyelids; bloody urine			Low back pain due to degenerative spinal disc 500 mg to 5 g daily	
(Severe late scurvy)			Air pollution ("smog") 3 g per day, with vitamins E and A	
Dingy and brownish complexion; severe weakness, the slightest exertion causes palpitation and breathlessness; spongy and bleeding gums; teeth become loose and may fall out; jawbone rots; extremely foul breath; old wounds may break open, fresh wounds won't heal; severe pain in limbs; brittle bones; pneumonia; death from sudden collapse			Mental illness	
			Mild symptoms (fatigue, pessimistic, worried states) 3 g daily	
(Mental symptoms)			Moderate symptoms (anxiety, depression, confusion, insomnia, etc.) 3 to 10 g daily	
Fatigue, listlessness, lassitude, confusion, depression; haggard, frowning, "pained" expression on face with careworn, knitted brow			Nighttime sedation, 1 to 5 g at bedtime	
			Severe symptoms (severe depression, "nervous breakdown") 3 to 30 g daily	
			Heroin or other drug withdrawal Up to 50 g daily	

BIOFLAVINOIDS (VITAMIN P COMPLEX)
Use Only Under a Physician's Supervision

SYMPTOMS AND SIGNS OF DEFICIENCY	RECOMMENDED DAILY REQUIREMENT	THERAPEUTIC DOSAGE	RICH NATURAL SOURCES
Easy bruising	Unknown	Sedation and stimulation 50 mg daily	CITRUS FRUITS, APRICOTS, CHERRIES, GRAPES, GREEN PEPPERS, TOMATOES, PAPAYA, BROCCOLI, CANTALOUPE
		Preventing traumatic bruising	
		Habitual and threatened miscarriage	
		Recurrent nosebleeds	
		Excessive menstrual bleeding	
		Hemorrhoids	
		Asthma	
		Bleeding gums 50 mg three times daily	

The Fat-Soluble Vitamins: A, D, E, and K

Vitamins are of two types, fat soluble and water soluble. Fat-soluble vitamins dissolve in alcohol and are more easily stored in the body. Because the fat-soluble vitamins are more easily stored, great excesses of fat-soluble vitamins A, D, and E can produce toxicity. Vitamin toxicity is completely reversible if caught in time, leaving no permanent damage, by reduction of the excessive intake. Vitamin K has shown no evidence of toxicity even in large amounts. Synthetic forms of all the fat-soluble vitamins have been developed, and all are appreciably more toxic than the natural vitamin. Vitamin deficiency, however, is much more likely today than vitamin excess.

Vitamin A

Vitamin A is necessary to promote growth, prevent blindness, build new tissues, and protect against infection. Vitamin A exists in nature in two forms: a form present in plants, carotene (first isolated from carrots), and an animal form. Most of the vitamin A in our diet is in the carotene form, and our bodies convert it into usable vitamin A. Vitamin E aids the absorption of vitamin A.

A Case of Vitamin A Deficiency

Jerry from Sacramento believed he was so homely that the other students were laughing at him. Anxious and unable to concentrate, he fell far behind in his studies and finally stopped attending classes.

The otherwise handsome lad's face was badly marked by adolescent acne. Jerry was taking antibiotics twice daily to destroy the skin bacteria aggravating the acne.

Jerry's night vision was so poor that he no longer drove in the evening. The combination of acne plus night blindness prompted me to prescribe 50,000 IU of vitamin A from fish liver oil daily, along with zinc. In addition, he was placed on an anti-anxiety regimen of B and C vitamins, especially B_6.

A month later, his night vision had improved and his complexion was better. His vitamin A was reduced to a maintenance 25,000 IU daily. Convinced his cola drink diet and chain smoking were aggravating both his anxiety and his skin, he switched to a high-protein diet with plenty of fresh green vegetables. Jerry felt calmer and resumed his studies.

Nervous young men and women often develop oily skin and acne as one expression of anxiety. Stress lowers blood vitamin A levels, and vitamin A, along with zinc and B_6, often helps anxiety-induced acne.

Acne or bumpy skin and night blindness, as in Jerry's case, are symptoms of vitamin A deficiency; vitamin A protects the epithelial tissues of the skin and is essential to normal vision.

Vitamin A deficiency creates ideal conditions for bacterial growth and the development of acne. A person's skin is constantly exposed to millions of bacteria. If the diet is adequate in vitamin A, skin cells continuously secrete a mucus which cleanses the surface and prevents bacterial growth. During vitamin A deficiency, skin cells grow more rapidly than usual but die quickly. These cells are crowded forward by other rapidly growing cells which likewise die quickly until there accumulates a cheesylike surface of layer on layer of packed dead cells. Dead cells cannot secrete the protective mucus. They also provide the neessary food for bacterial growth, and the resulting acne.[1]

Using antibiotics to kill the bacteria is indirect treatment which doesn't touch one real cause of acne, the vitamin A deficiency. Some skin doctors now use vitamin A to treat acne. The vitamin A works slowly; it can take four months to show improvement, but it effectively treats the cause without harmful side effects. Antibiotics, in addition to killing the skin bacteria, also kill helpful intestinal bacteria which make several vitamins for us.

Eyes that tire or ache from reading or close work, burning and itching eyes, inflamed eyelids, headache, and eyeball pain can all signify vitamin A deficiency. Severe and prolonged deficiency leads to xerophthalmia, a major source of blindness in children of malnourished areas of the world.

Winter inceases the need for vitamin A, as the body metabolizes it more slowly in cold weather. This may explain why children grow faster in the summertime, since vitamin A promotes growth. It proves Mom's common sense nutritional wisdom when she insisted I take my vitamin A-rich cod liver oil while we endured the hard Dakota winters.

Why should the body require more vitamin A during cold weather? Vitamin A stimulates the body's adrenal and thyroid glands, which maintain the body's metabolism, producing heat and fostering growth. Not only does vitamin A spur these glands but, by a feedback mechanism, increased activity of these glands stimulates the availability of vitamin A. Thus vitamin A stores in the liver are depleted when the thyroid is underactive. Thyroid appears necessary to convert carotene (the plant precursor) into usable vitamin A.[2]

These glands, along with the thymus, the body's "organ of immunity," also protect us from infectious illness. Vitamin A feeds them all. Frequent colds, sinus trouble, pneumonia, and other respiratory troubles may signal vitamin A deficiency. Vitamin A deficiency also reduces the number of white blood cells, the body's infection fighters. Herein too is one possible reason why diabetics are so susceptible to infections. Diabetics, along with hypothyroids, cannot use beta-carotene, the common form of vitamin A in our diet. Diabetics *can* use animal form vitamin A, the type found in fish liver oil, egg yolk, milk fat, and organ meats, especially liver. There is hardly any vitamin A in pork or beefsteak.

Old age and disease, especially liver and intestinal disease, decrease the body's ability to transform plant carotene into usable vitamin A.

Vitamin A works with protein to promote growth and build healthy tissues. When vitamin A (or protein) is deficient, hair lacks luster and sheen, dandruff accumulates on the scalp, and nails peel easily or become ridged. "Goose bumps" at the site of the hair follicles may appear on the skin in vitamin A deficiency.

Sexual disorders in both sexes have been attributed to vitamin A deficiency, as well as birth defects (cleft palate, congenital defects of the eye and heart) and calcium phosphate-type kidney stones.

Vitamin A and Mental Illness

Insomnia, fatigue, depression, and nerve pains in the extremities may be signs of vitamin A deficiency.

Vitamin A levels do decrease under stress, and vitamin A is needed in the manufacture of "antistress" adrenal hormones. Therefore, I prescribe a 25,000 IU vitamin A supplement (from fish liver oil) for anxious patients.

In one type of mental illness, anorexia nervosa, the beta-carotene form of vitamin A is markedly *elevated* in the bloodstream.[3] In anorexia nervosa the patient loses his appetite and takes so little food that he becomes severely emaciated. Since lack of appetite (anorexia) is a symptom of excessive vitamin A, the finding of excessive beta-carotene (the plant precursor of vitamin A) in the blood of patients with anorexia nervosa would seem to have tremendous significance.

Lowering High Cholesterol with Vitamin A

One hundred thousand units of vitamin A acetate for four to six months lowered cholesterol levels in persons with high cholesterol and hardening of the arteries but had no effect on persons with normal cholesterol levels.[4]

Vitamin A Toxicity

Naomi, a nutrition-conscious woman in her mid-thirties, consulted me, puzzled.

"I can't understand it. I'm careful about my diet, take all my supplements, don't eat junk food—but still I have trouble. I'm losing my hair, my lips are cracking and my skin is dry, but it *can't* be a B vitamin deficiency. I've been taking a high-potency B-complex every day for years.

"I've been feeling irritable and depressed for months now," she continued. "I have zero appetite, but I keep eating because I know I must. I get aches and pains and have this terrible headache which won't go away!"

"Can you describe what the headache is like?" I requested.

"It's a pressure feeling, as if it's too full inside and my head is going to explode."

"Would one of your supplements be vitamin A?" I questioned.

"Yes," she replied. "I have bad skin and take vitamin A to keep it in check."

"How much do you take?"

"I take 100,000 units a day, and have been for several months."

Naomi's skin was yellow, and when I felt her belly, I found her liver and spleen were enlarged.

"Please stop the vitamin A immediately. Take this lab slip and we will measure the vitamin A level in your blood."

At her next visit, obviously in better health, she confided, "I must have been poisoning myself with the vitamin A. A few days after I stopped, my headache went away and my appetite returned; I'm no longer losing my hair and I feel one thousand percent better."

Her blood vitamin A level was 545 IU per 100 ml (80 to 300 is normal), confirming the vitamin A toxicity.

Vitamin A is soluble in fat and is retained and stored in the body, whereas excesses of the water-soluble vitamins B and C pass out harmlessly in the urine. Almost 95% of the body's vitamin A is stored in the liver, which holds about 600,000 IU. Excesses of vitamin A therefore swell the liver and disturb its function. Naomi's poor appetite and yellow skin were due to either the disturbed liver function or the excess of vitamin A itself. The type of vitamin A found in plants, beta-carotene, in excess in the body causes a yellowing of the skin, carotenemia. A friend of mine developed carotenemia when she ate armloads of carrots while kicking cigarettes. Carotenemia is harmless and can be distinguished from the yellowing of liver disease (jaundice), because the whites of the eyes turn yellow in liver disease but not in carotenemia.

Excessive vitamin A increases the fluid pressure in the brain, causing swelling which produced Naomi's headaches and sensation of fullness. If severe, this swelling can be fatal. A young mother read in Adelle Davis that a person should take 25,000 units of vitamin A daily. Misunderstanding this recommendation, the mother gave 25,000 units of vitamin A daily to her infant, a greatly excessive dose for the baby. The cranial bones of newborn babies are still soft, and this toxic dose caused swelling of the brain fluid resulting in separation of the bones of the skull and expansion of the head. The infant was near death before the mother's mistake was discovered. Fortunately, vitamin A overdose is completely reversible by discontinuing the vitamin, and the baby recovered from its accidental poisoning.

Weight loss, dry and atrophied skin, hair loss, sore eyes, decalcification and spontaneous fracture of bones, irritability, depression, cracks in the lips, and thickening of the bones are all possible signs of vitamin A toxicity.

Vitamin A and Cancer

Dr. Michael B. Sporn[5] of the National Cancer Institute proposes that vitamin A and substances chemically related to vitamin A (analogs) can make important contributions to the prevention of cancer. More than half of all human cancer starts in epithelial tissue. Epithelial tissue forms the lining of organs and glands such as mammary glands, skin, and passages in the body. The lungs, gut, bladder, and reproductive organs are all lined with this epithelial tissue. The epithelial tissue depends on vitamin A for its normal development. Without sufficient vitamin A, these epithelial cells often undergo precancerous changes. Laboratory studies demonstrate that animals deficient in vitamin A have increased vulnerability to cancer-causing chemicals (carcinogens). Vitamin A protects animals given such chemicals from stomach, lung, respiratory, and uterine cancer. A recent study of over 8000 Norwegian men demonstrated a diet adequate in vitamin A significantly reduces smokers' chances of developing lung cancer. Further, vitamin A and some closely related substances can actually *reverse* precancerous changes in cells of the prostate gland.

Obtaining Vitamin A

The plant form of A (beta-carotene) is richly present in green leafy vegetables, such as spinach, broccoli, and alfalfa, in yellow tubers like carrots, and in fruits. One carrot contains 11,000 IU of carotene.

The widespread use of commercial fertilizers threatens this vegetable vitamin A source. High in nitrogen, these fertilizers develop nitrites which interfere with the body's ability to convert plant carotene into usable vitamin A. The longer plant foods are stored, the more nitrates convert to nitrites. These same nitrites are used to preserve and color all types of processed, canned, and cured meats (sausages, bologna, salami, and franks). Ozone and nitrogen dioxide air pollutants use up vitamin A, as does smoking.

Cod liver oil, one teaspoon daily in the winter months, or lightly cooked beef or chicken liver are good natural sources. A half-pound of calf's liver contains about 74,000 IU of vitamin A. If you suspect a deficiency, the cheapest available vitamin A capsules from fish liver oil are best. Since the liver stores A for up to three months, it is not necessary to supplement daily. Fish liver oil is preferable to synthetic vitamin A as, dose for dose, synthetic vitamin A is more likely to cause toxicity. While an adult can take 25,000 units daily indefinitely with safety, an infant or a child, because of small body weight, cannot. Cod liver oil as a source of vitamin A is more satisfactory for chilren and is available in mint and cherry flavors.

Department of Agriculture recommended daily allowances of vitamin A are 1500 IU for infants, 3000 IU for children up to twelve, and 6000 IU for adults. Nationwide studies by the Department of Agriculture reveal one person in four gets less than 5000 IU of vitamin A daily.

Vitamin D

Vitamin D inceases calcium and phosphate absorption from the gut and is necessary for normal bone development. Vitamin D, by increasing calcium absorption and favoring its retention and utilization by the body, can indirectly affect the mind. Adequate calcium is needed to relax nerves, induce sound sleep, and decrease sensitivity to pain.

Vitamin D may be particularly needed by women during menopause, when calcium intake is usually low. I sometimes find calcium and vitamin D effective in treating the hot flashes, night sweats, leg cramps, irritability, nervousness, and depression of a woman's change of life.

Vitamin D Deficiency

Lack of vitamin D leads to inadequate absorption of calcium from the gut and retention of phosphorus in the kidney, causing faulty mineralization of the bones. The bones become soft (osteomalacia), and the victim experiences rheumatic pains and exhaustion. If severe, the condition is fatal.

In children, vitamin D deficiency (rickets) is not uncommon in sunlight-deprived urban areas, where pollution blocks the sun. Sunlight makes vitamin D by acting on oils on the skin. Adding synthetic vitamin D (D_2) to milk and milk products to prevent such deficiency is now a widespread practice.

Synthetic D_2 Toxicity?

Because dairy products have been supplemented with synthetic irradiated ergosterol (vitamin D_2), rickets is now rare in the United States, but hardening of the arteries (atherosclerosis) is increasing. A few scientists think the increase may be due to excessive irradiated ergosterol (synthetic vitamin D_2) in your diet.[6]

Milk as it comes from the cow (raw milk) contains about 25 units of natural vitamin D (D_3) per quart. Since the heating process of pasteurization largely destroys natural D_3, synthetic vitamin D_2 (irradiated ergosterol) is added. The 400 units of irradiated ergosterol added per quart is roughly sixteen times as much as was originally present. Vitamin D acts to lay down calcium in tissues. Since the addition of irradiated ergosterol (D_2) to foods, the incidence of hypercalcium diseases (calciphylaxis) has become more frequent. Hans Selye in his book *Calciphylaxis*[7] first called attention to the occurrence in industrialized nations of several hundred clinical conditions associated with abnormal calcium deposits. Calcium deposits in the arteries of even young children are now a common finding. In Sweden, recent reports reveal pathologic calcium deposits in the arteries of nearly every infant autopsied.[8] "Prophylactic" levels of vitamin D_2 added to foods may be responsible for this alarming finding.

Natural vitamin D is less likely to cause this pathologic calcification of the soft tissues of the body. Pathologic calcification due to vitamin D toxicity can also be prevented by the simultaneous use of generous amounts of vitamins C, E, and/or the B vitamin choline. Deficiencies of vitamin E or magnesium make calciphylaxis more likely. Pathologic calcification has been implicated in some cases of mental retardation.

Vitamin D and Dr. Carl Reich

Dr. Reich is a Canadian physician who has been using large doses of vitamin D along with vitamin A to treat a number of conditions which he labels "spastic conduit diseases."[9] Included are some forms of chronic asthma and arthritis, as well as many states of chronic anxiety and depression. Dr. Reich believes these conditions are due to a long-standing calcium deficiency. He gives modest calcium supplements, along with sizeable doses of natural vitamin A (up to 60,000 IU) and natural vitamin D (up to 6000 units) daily. He has used these levels for three to six months on thousands of patients without evidence of toxicity.

Severe muscle spasm, especially of the neck and shoulders, is certainly a common problem. It is almost an inevitable accompaniment of anxiety states. If megadoses of vitamin A and D are helpful, it would be a great boon.

Obtaining Vitamin D

Vitamin D is called the "sunshine" vitamin because it is formed by the sun's rays acting on the oils of the skin. This is one argument against too frequent or vigorous bathing, as hot soapy baths wash away the oils needed to form vitamin D. We can also obtain vitamin D from egg yolk, liver, and fish. Three and one-half ounces of sardines, herring, or salmon provide the daily requirement.

The National Research Council has set the dietary allowance of vitamin D at 400 IU per day for infants and adults. Sufficient exposure to sunlight meets most of this need.

Vitamin D supplements may be desirable during the winter to help prevent colds. I recommend that vitamin D be given with vitamin A in the natural form from fish liver oil. Capsules containing 10,000 IU of vitamin A and 400 IU of vitamin D or 25,000 IU of vitamin A and 1000 IU of vitamin D are available at health food stores. High potency Norwegian cod liver oil is also available from health food or drug stores. For equivalent potencies, cod liver oil is least expensive and most desirable if you don't mind the taste. One tablespoon of high potency Norwegian cod liver oil contains 35,000 IU of vitamin A and 3500 IU of vitamin D. This provides a concentrated means of obtaining Dr. Reich's megadoses for the treatment of chronic anxiety, depression, asthma, and arthritis. Because of the risk of toxicity, such treatment should occur only under a physician's supervision.

Vitamin E (Tocopherol)

The word tocopherol is a combination of the Greek *tokos*, meaning childbirth, with the word *phero*, meaning to bear, thus, "to bear children." The discoverer of tocopherol found that male rats deprived of vitamin E became sterile, whereas female rats so deprived were unable to conceive. If given vitamin E but an insufficient amount, they would conceive but were unable to carry the fetus to full term and live birth. From these early observations, vitamin E has earned a generous reputation as an aphrodisiac (see Chapter 11).

Vitamin E is found in the oils of all grains, nuts, and seeds. Except for alpha-tocopherol (there are four identified tocopherols: alpha, beta, gamma, and delta), it is lost during exposure to air, heating, freezing, and storage. Frying foods in oil, for example, destroys 75% of it. Essentially none remains in typical "supermarket" refined oils, or in refined flour and packaged cereals.

Vitamin E and the Mind

Vitamin E normally is found in the brain and other vital organs, especially the sex, adrenal, and pituitary glands; their good function is essential for mental as well as physical health. Therefore, vitmain E has a subtle, salubrious effect on nervous or exhausted individuals. German researchers, first noticing vitamin E's calming effect, dubbed it "Nature's own tranquilizer."

In 1950, Dr. N. R. Kavinoky[10] reported that vitamin E helped relieve the symptoms of menopause. Nervousness, fatigue, restless sleep, and insomnia were reduced in more than half of a group of seventy-nine patients, while nearly all the patients suffering heart palpitation, dizziness, and shortness of breath were relieved within two weeks to three months.

Vitamin E and Polyunsaturated Oils

Vitamin E functions as an anti-oxidant, preventing unsaturated fatty acids and fatlike substances from being destroyed by oxygen. Excessive oxygen turns polyunsaturated fats in the body's cells rancid (peroxidation) unless sufficient vitamin E is present to prevent this. Polyunsaturated fats are the types found in safflower and corn oil. Though originally containing adequate vitamin E to prevent this peroxidation, these unsaturated oils have lost nearly all their vitamin E in processing. Vegetable oils, unless designated as unrefined, are extracted by chemicals and high heat. They are bleached, refined to neutralize the free fatty acids, and, most disastrously, "deodorized" by being boiled for up to twelve hours. Any vitamin E remaining is purely accidental. This is the polyunsaturated oil which many physicians recommend in place of saturated (animal) fats and cholesterol in preventing heart disease.

Free Radicals

Not only oxygen but also the common air pollutants ozone and nitrous oxide, as well as the sun's rays, x-rays, and any type of ionizing radiation, can knock loose a hydrogen atom and cause this peroxidation of polyunsaturated lipids. When this happens, free radicals are formed.

The free radical flies about within the cell under terrific force and without any pattern to its movement until it strikes another molecule and causes damage. Constant and increasing free radical damage may be involved in the creation of cancers. Vitamin E guards against the formation of these dangerous free radicals.

Increasing free radical damage is one theory of the cause of aging. Vitamin E may therefore prolong youth. By adding vitamin E to a test-tube culture of human cells at ten times the level normally found in human tissue, Drs. L. Packer and J. R. Smith more than doubled the life span of human cells.[11]

In conditions of poor intestinal absorption, such as celiac disease, sprue, and cystic fibrosis, vitamin E deficiency can occur, causing degeneration and death of nerve and muscle cells. Vitamin E deficiency also causes anemia in premature infants due to increased destruction of blood cells, just as occurs in animals made deficient experimentally. When animals are fed processed polyunsaturated fats, their stores of vitamin E are quickly consumed. Once the protective E is exhausted, the polyunsaturates undergo the peroxidation process, liberating free radicals. The free radicals wreak cellular havoc, causing destruction and death of nerve, muscle, and blood cells.

Consuming unsaturated fats without vitamin E may therefore actually be hastening our demise. One group of experimental animals[12] was fed heated polyunsaturates in the form of corn oil. Another group was fed heated butter. Those fed heated corn oil suffered from diarrhea, grew less, had rough fur, and all developed tumors, only one surviving the forty-month period of the experiment. None of the rats fed heated butter got tumors, and all of them survived.

If you use polyunsaturated "supermarket" oils, take 200 IU of vitamin E daily to prevent formation of free radicals. Or use only cold-pressed vegetable oil or "virgin" olive oil which still retains its vitamin E.

Vitamin E and Heart Disease

Heart disease, from coronary thrombosis, kills over a million people a year in the United States alone. At the turn of the century, bread still contained wheat germ, with its vitamin E-rich oil. People used eggs, cream, and butter liberally, all high in cholesterol, but coronary thrombosis was unheard of. In the past fifteen years, the American intake of animal fat has been reduced by two-thirds, yet the coronary rate until recently has climbed steadily every year. The declining amounts of vitamin E in the diet have correlated inversely with this generally rising heart attack rate. Before wheat germ was discarded by machine milling and further vitamin E destroyed by the bleaching of flour, a typical American diet contained about 150 IU of vitamin E. By 1960 this amount had declined precipitously to 15 IU, and today the average diet contains only 7.4 IU.

Recently there has been a slight decrease in coronary disease, probably because Americans now get more exercise and are paying more attention to their diet. It has been estimated that 35 million Americans are now taking supplements of vitamin E.[13]

Vitamin E and Oxygen

Russian athletes take vitamin E for its oxygen-sparing effect. Their researchers consider 100 to 150 IU optimal for training periods of one-and-a-half to two hours.

In the 1960s our early space astronauts would return to Earth anemic and exhausted. Dr. David Turner recognized the astronauts were breathing oxygen-rich air, and the oxygen was depleting their vitamin E reserves, leading to destruction of blood cells and subsequent anemia. Vitamin E supplements solved the astronauts' problem.

Windfield Farm racehorses in Toronto, Canada, were given vitamin E, with the resultant number of wins per horse jumping by as much as 66% in the first year supplementation was used. With the vitamin E these racehorses, many of which were notoriously high-strung and refused to eat properly, gradually quieted down and began eating normally.

Vitamin E is also used to heal burns and to prevent scarring. It is protective for women on the "pill." Women on birth control pills have a higher risk of thrombophlebitis (inflamed blood clotting of veins), perhaps because the estrogen in the pill uses up vitamin E. Thyroid and iron salts also antagonize vitamin E. Persons taking iron should do so at breakfast and lunch, and save their vitamin E for evening.

Vitamin E may be especially useful to city smog sufferers, as it protects against the damage caused by ozone and nitrogen oxide, two of the main toxins in polluted air.

Obtaining Vitamin E

I take 200 IU of mixed-tocopherols vitamin E daily, and recommend the natural mixed tocopherols over the synthetic d-alpha tocopherol as a matter of philosophy. D-alpha, though the most potent fraction, is only a fraction of the tocopherols found in nature and may not in itself perform the full spectrum of vitamin E's biological activity. Be careful that the vitamin E is fully potent, for unless it is carefully extracted it will lose its biological activity. Purchase reputable brand names and avoid private-label "sale" vitamins.

For smoggy air, severe physical exertion, x-rays, or even excessive exposure to the sun, I take 200 IU of mixed tocopherols three times a day. Though very large doses have been taken without harm, high levels can raise blood pressure, so I never exceed 600 IU daily unless using vitamin E therapeutically. Even then I never exceed 1600 IU a day.

Rich natural sources of vitamin E are wheat germ oil, cotton-seed oil, and safflower oil, but *only* if these oils are

Table 3

THE FAT-SOLUBLE VITAMINS.

Use Only Under a Physician's Guidance

FAT-SOLUBLE VITAMINS	SYMPTOMS AND SIGNS OF DEFICIENCY	SYMPTOMS OF TOXICITY	RECOMMENDED DAILY REQUIREMENT	SUPPLE- MENTAL DOSAGE	THERA- PEUTIC DOSAGE	RICH NATURAL SOURCES
VITAMIN A	Acne; bumpy skin; night blindness; achy, tired, burning, itching eyes; inflamed eyelids; headaches; eyeball pain; xerophthalmia; frequent colds; sinus trouble; recurrent respiratory illness. Dull, lusterless hair, ridged nails that peel easily, sexual disorders, birth defects; calcium phosphate kidney stones; precancerous changes in body tissues; mental changes—insomnia, fatigue, depression; nerve pains in the extremities	Mental symptoms—irritability and depression; aches and pains, poor appetite, hair loss, cracked lips, dry skin, yellowing of skin (carotenemia), enlarged liver, headaches, weight loss, sore eyes, decalcification and spontaneous fracture of bones, thickening of bones	Infants: 1500 IU Children: 3000 IU Adults: 6000 IU	10,000 IU daily, in fish liver oil	25,000 to 100,000 IU	PLANT FORM (beta-carotene) in GREEN LEAFY VEGETABLES (SPINACH, BROCCOLI, ALFALFA), YELLOW TUBERS (CARROTS), FRUITS, COD LIVER OIL, BEEF AND CHICKEN LIVER
VITAMIN D	"Soft bones" (rickets), rheumatic pains and exhaustion, menopausal symptoms, hypothyroidism	Calcification of body's soft tissues; increased frequency of urination, loss of appetite, nausea, vomiting, diarrhea, muscular weakness, dizziness, weariness	400 IU	One teaspoon cod liver oil in winter	1500 to 2800 IU from natural fish liver oil	COD LIVER OIL, SUNLIGHT

Vitamin	Deficiency symptoms	Toxicity / Notes	Recommended dosage			Food sources
VITAMIN E	Menopausal symptoms, restlessness, fatigue, fitful sleep, insomnia; increased destruction of red blood cells, muscle wasting, increased demand for oxygen, poor glandular function, liver and kidney damage	High blood pressure	Infants: 5 IU Children: 10 IU Adults: 15 IU	200 to 600 IU for adults	600 to 2000 IU for adults	WHEAT GERM OIL, COTTONSEED OIL, SAFFLOWER OIL (but only if cold-pressed), CABBAGE, SPINACH, ASPARAGUS, BROCCOLI, WHOLE GRAIN WHEAT, RICE, OATS, PEANUTS
VITAMIN K	Bleeding disorders	Synthetic vitamin K can damage the infant liver; natural vitamin K is not toxic	300 to 500 micrograms obtained in diet	Usually unnecessary	200 to 1600 micrograms	NORMAL INTESTINAL BACTERIAL FLORA, LEAFY GREEN VEGETABLES, TOMATOES, PORK LIVER, LEAN MEAT, PEAS, CARROTS, SOYBEANS, POTATOES

cold-pressed, as is Viobin brand wheat germ oil. Cabbage, spinach, asparagus, and broccoli are good vegetable sources, and whole grain wheat, rice, oats, and peanuts also have ample vitamin E.

Vitamin K

Vitamin K, discovered in Denmark by a man named Dam, is a yellow oil manufactured by our intestinal bacteria and present richly in leafy green vegetables (spinach, cabbage, kale, and cauliflower). Vitamin K deficiency or excess manifests no known effect on the mind. Vitamin K's function is to assist in blood clotting; thus its name K, from "Koagulation," the Danish spelling of "coagulation."

Newborns receiving a low K diet, suffering from diarrhea, or on bacteria-destroying antibiotics risk vitamin K deficiency leading to bleeding problems. A bad liver interferes with the use of vitamin K in making prothrombin, the clotting factor. The elderly, because of poor diet and frequent antibiotic therapy, are particularly likely to be vitamin K deficient. Excessive menstrual flow in women can signify deficiency.

Obtaining Vitamin K

Most of us need not supplement our diet with vitamin K if we eat leafy green vegetables, tomatoes, pork liver, lean meat, peas, carrots, soybeans, and potatoes.

Natural vitamin K is not toxic, even when taken in huge amounts, but synthetic K can damage an infant's liver.

Since our intestinal bacteria make some vitamin K and perhaps all the B vitamins, it is important to maintain a healthy intestinal flora. Intestinal illness or the use of bacteria-destroying antibiotics may cause the replacement of the normal gut flora by unhealthy putrefactive bacteria. These bacteria may cause diarrhea, rectal itching, excessive passing of gas, or foul-smelling stools. The normal flora can be restored by drinking acidophilus culture with every meal for a few weeks. Available in health food stores, it has a fizzy, effervescent taste. Tablets of a mixed culture of *Lactobacillus acidophilus* and *Lactobacillus bulgaricus* (Lactinex®) are available at drug stores with a doctor's prescription. Eating copious amounts of yogurt containing the living bacterial culture will also help restore the correct flora.

The fat-soluble vitamins are vitally important to physical and mental health. Like other nutrients, they can be most reliably obtained by using unprocessed natural oils and fats. Butter, for example, though maligned in recent years as "animal fat," retains its vitamin E, while margarine, though trouted as a "health spread," is highly processed and contains additives.

Polyunsaturated vegetable oils, if they are cold-pressed "virgin" oils, are an excellent source of vitamin E as well as the essential fatty acids (vitamin F), important to the nerves and brain. Animal fats (liver, butter, cheese) provide fat-soluble vitamins A and D. The natural forms of the fat-soluble vitamins, as opposed to the synthetic, present a lesser risk of toxicity.

The Elements:
Part One—
The Bulk Minerals

In the sweat of thy face shalt thou eat bread, till thou return unto the ground; for out of it wast thou taken; for dust thou art, and unto dust shalt thou return.

—GENESIS

The elements are a class of substances, 103 of which have now been identified, which cannot be chemically separated into simpler substances. They are the basic particles of which all matter, including our bodies, is composed.

The major elements of the human body are the organic elements, oxygen, carbon, hydrogen, and nitrogen, which form organic compounds in the body. We are 65% oxygen, 18% carbon, and 10% hydrogen, all of which are supplied by our food, water, and air. Our 3% nitrogen comes from protein. About 90% of our oxygen is combined with 7% of our hydrogen to form water (H_2O), comprising roughly two-thirds of our body weight.

The other elements of which we are composed are the inorganic minerals calcium (1.5%), phosphorus (1%), potassium (0.35%), sulfur (0.25%), sodium (0.15%), chlorine (0.15%), magnesium (0.05%), and silicon (0.05%). These elements are known as the *bulk minerals*. Sulfur and phosphorus participate with the remaining oxygen and hydrogen, along with carbon and nitrogen, to form the body's organic compounds, the carbohydrates, fats, proteins, etc., which comprise 90% of the body's solid matter.

Minerals resemble vitamins in that they supply no calories to the body, though they are vital for life. Humans can tolerate a deficiency of vitamins longer than a deficiency of minerals. A slight change in the blood's level of important minerals may rapidly endanger health and survival.[1] Minerals like sodium, potassium, and chloride help regulate the body fluids and maintain our correct balance of acids and bases.

Plants and animals can manufacture vitamins but not minerals; if the mineral isn't in the soil, it won't be in the plant. Much of our soil has been drained of minerals because of continuous plantings and the use of commercial synthetic fertilizers. Synthetic fertilizers usually provide only nitrogen, phosphorus, and potassium because these elements have the largest impact on plant growth. With continuous use of commercial fertilizers, which replace only three elements, the soil becomes depleted in other minerals which are equally important for good human nutrition. Foods grown in such mineral-depleted soil become depleted and imbalanced in minerals. Refining foods inevitably removes most of the remaining minerals. Since refined foods and foods grown with commercial fertilizers may be deficient or imbalanced in minerals, organically grown unrefined foods are best to assure an adequate mineral supply.

All minerals, as well as other nutrients, appear to have specific effects on the mind; I use them extensively in my practice and measure the body's levels of important minerals in nearly every patient. In this chapter we consider the bulk minerals and their action on the mind; in Chapter 7, we study the essential trace minerals and in Chapter 8 the toxic minerals.

Calcium (Ca)

Calcium is the most abundant mineral in the body. Adults contain about three pounds of calcium, accounting for over 2% of total body weight. Foods high in oxalic acid (spinach, rhubarb, chocolate), cereal grains, excessive fats, and phosphates in the diet all interfere with calcium absorption in the gut by forming insoluble calcium salts and indigestible calcium soaps. On the other hand, vitamins A, D, and C all facilitate the absorption of calcium. Calcium in the diet probably aids in the absorption of vitamin B_{12}.

Calcium and the Mind

Ninety-nine percent of our body calcium is present in the bones and teeth. It is the other 1%, present in the soft tissues and blood, which crucially affects the nerves. Extreme calcium deficiency (tetany) causes muscle twitchings, cramps, confusion, irritation, and spasm of the throat, with labored breathing and convulsions. Tetany is very rare, but I commonly see less severe but nevertheless significant calcium lack. The U.S. Department of Agriculture estimated in 1968 that over 30% of Americans are calcium-deficient. Such calcium shortage may result in a grouchy, irritable, tense disposition, with depression, impairment of memory, insomnia, and cramping in the calves.

Anxiety Attacks and Calcium Deficiency

There are strong similarities between the symptoms of an anxiety attack and the mental symptoms of calcium deficiency. Doctors administered lactic acid, under double-blind conditions, to two groups, one comprised of normal subjects and the other patients suffering anxiety. In some cases, calcium ions were added to the lactic acid, forming a compound called calcium lactate. Lactic acid alone precipitated anxiety attacks in thirteen out of fourteen of the anxious subjects within a minute or two after the infusion was started, and also in two of the ten normal control subjects. But when calcium lactate was used, anxiety symptoms for the most part didn't occur. This experiment has two important implications. First, it demonstrates a biochemical cause for anxiety, lactic acid; second, it indicates that calcium in sufficient quantities will prevent anxiety attacks.[2]

Further evidence that adequate body calcium promotes mental well-being is provided by Dr. F. Flack, who has discovered that improvement in depression is accompanied by increased retention of calcium in the body.[3]

Anxious individuals frequently hyperventilate. Such rapid deep breathing causes an alkalosis (increased blood bicarbonate) which lowers the level of active calcium in the bloodstream. The resulting calcium deficiency induces confusion, dizziness, numbness, and muscle cramps.

Often calcium-deficient patients complain that they feel as if they're dying; in fact, calcium and associated phosphorus in abundant amounts help keep us young. Prematurely old persons have lower blood levels of calcium and phosphorus and x-ray evidence of mineral loss in their bones (osteoporosis).[4]

Calcium and Allergies

Allergy sufferers are often benefited by calcium supplements, perhaps because calcium lowers histamine and excessive histamine causes the allergic reaction. Dr. Alice Bernheim relieved allergy symptoms in 80% of thirty chronic cases by using calcium, plus other measures to aid calcium absorption.[5] Eight of her patients previously had taken calcium alone without effect. Dr. Bernheim administered calcium in the proper manner to assure maximum absorption, that is, between meals, along with vitamin D and hydrochloric acid and/or lactose to provide acid. One of the cases completely relieved of all symptoms for the first time was an asthmatic, with severe eczema and hayfever.

Calcium Interactions

Birth control pills lower blood calcium and zinc and raise blood copper and iron.[6]

Bodies depleted of calcium and the other essential minerals are sitting ducks for the invasion of the toxic metals lead, cadmium, and mercury, while abundant body calcium and other minerals discourage the uptake of toxic metals as well as radioactive strontium-90. I use calcium supplements with other minerals to treat lead, mercury, or cadmium toxicity.

Researchers credit the English habit of taking milk with tea as the reason English tea drinkers have a much lower rate of bladder cancer compared with Indian tea drinkers who take it plain. Tannic acid, the substance in tea and red wine which leaves a "furry" feeling on your palate, is used to tan leather and can have a similar effect on your kidneys. Calcium in the milk attaches to the tannic acid in tea, detoxifying it.

The kidneys reabsorb some of the calcium and magnesium passed out in the urine, but sugar in the diet inhibits this mineral-saving mechanism. A high-sugar diet thus plays a significant role in calcium loss and softening of the bones (osteomalacia).[7] Chocolate also lowers calcium and phospohorus levels in rats,[8] so offering chocolate milk to induce children to drink their calcium might be self-defeating.

Obtaining Calcium

Milk and dairy products are the best sources for calcium, an eight-ounce glass of milk providing 30% of the daily calcium requirement, well-balanced with magnesium and phosphorus. In addition to calcium and magnesium, milk is also rich in tryptophan, all three of which sedate the brain, explaining why a glass of warm milk at bedtime remedies sleeplessness. However, milk contains lactose sugar which 70% of adult Blacks and 6% of adult Whites do not tolerate.[9] In such susceptible individuals, milk causes flatulence, belching, stomach cramps, and a watery diarrhea. Though lactose normally improves the absorption of calcium and phosphorus, in lactose-intolerant individuals it increases calcium loss in the feces.

Molasses and vegetables like peas, beans, potatoes, cauliflower, and dried figs supply calcium, as does hard water.

Dolomite and bone meal are excellent inexpensive supplements for both calcium and magnesium, though both suffer from possible lead contamination. Dolomite is mined in open pits and subject to atmospheric lead fallout. Lead is taken up, along with strontium-90, and stored in animal bones, leading to contaminated bone meal.

Calcium lactate, calcium gluconate, and calcium chloride are all available supplements. A gram a day is the recommended adult dose; pregnant and nursing women need a gram and a half. Exposure to sunlight and formation of vitamin D increase calcium absorption and the daily requirement may be reduced.

Magnesium (Mg)

The magnesium in our body weighs a little less than one ounce, amounting to five-hundreths of a percent of the body's content. Provided the soil they were grown in is adequate in magnesium, many foods offer good sources of the mineral, especially green vegetables. Many soils, especially in the South, are now deficient in magnesium. Soil deficiences of iron, zinc, manganese, and calcium are also widespread.

Magnesium maintains vital body balances with sodium and chloride and calcium and phosphorus. It is required by protein and carbohydrate metabolism, and involved in the heart, kidney, and bones, which contain 66% of our magnesium. Magnesium is a natural tranquilizer for the nervous system, and I use it extensively in my practice.

Alcohol Promotes Magnesium Depletion

Ever wonder why excessive drinking produces a hangover? Alcohol generates a loss of body water and thus of water-soluble vitamins and many minerals, chiefly magnesium. All the common hangover symptoms—sensitivity to sounds, twitching, tremors, dizziness, rapid heartbeat, aching muscles, fatigue, depression, and grouchiness—are also typical symptoms of magnesium deficiency. Other nutrient deficiencies can also induce such symptoms, and vitamin B_1 (thiamine) loss is partly responsible for alcoholic hangover. But thiamine deficiency cannot be corrected with thiamine alone unless sufficient magnesium is present in the body; so I always give alcoholics thiamine and magnesium.

Treating Nervousness with Magnesium

Because of its calming effect on the nervous system, I commonly employ magnesium in treating anxiety, depression, insomnia, and hyperactivity in children.

In a study of suicide statistics, French scientist M. L. Robinet discovered that "the comparison of geological maps and statistics establishes in a striking manner the influence of the magnesium content of the soil on the number of suicides. ... It is evident that one doesn't commit suicide because the soil is poor in magnesium. But, those who regularly absorbed a good amount of magnesium salts have a more stable equilibrium, they support adversity with more calm and do not renounce everything to avoid some sorrow.... The use of magnesium permits one to support adversity with more serenity."

Total body magnesium is low in psychiatric depression and increases with recovery.[10] Magnesium levels in the blood plasma remain normal, but the magnesium in the cells decreases in depression, and it is this intracellular magnesium deficiency which is responsible for the symptoms.[11]

Many insomniacs harbor a magnesium deficiency; it is magnesium deficiency which probably explains why alcoholics are such poor sleepers.

Birth control pills decrease serum magnesium levels. Magnesium is at its lowest in women during the menstrual period. Many women feel blue with the onset of menses ("the weeping of the womb"), and the lowered magnesium level provides a biochemical explanation.

To hyperactive children I give magnesium supplements and insist they eat green vegetables to increase magnesium in the diet. Epileptics sometimes benefit from magnesium's quieting effect, which reduces the likelihood of seizures; and magnesium can be helpful for infantile convulsions.

Severe magnesium deficiency can even induce visual hallucinations, delirium, confusion, and seizures, as seen in alcoholic withdrawal (delirium tremens). These symptoms may be partly due to an associated calcium depletion, as a person low in magnesium cannot absorb adequate calcium.

Magnesium Deficiency and the Body

Low body magnesium may precipitate *kidney stones,* and magnesium salts with vitamin B_6 (pyridoxine) will prevent stones in those prone to them. Magnesium deficiency in both the plasma and the cells is seen in *high blood pressure,*[12] and since magnesium dilates blood vessels, it has been suggested as a therapy for hypertension. Drugs which lower the blood pressure also raise cellular magnesium levels.[13] Magnesium in the heart muscle is decreased in persons dying of sudden *heart attacks* or from long-standing coronary insufficiency.

In summary, magnesium deficiency seems related to many of our common diseases; and magnesium is in short supply in our Western diet. Dr. Mildred Seelig[14] reports there is almost twice as much magnesium per ounce of food in the Oriental diet as in ours. The Western diet is high in protein, calcium, and vitamin D, and alcohol use is common, all of which increase our magnesium requirement The average diet's daily magnesium (250 to 300 mg) should be doubled, suggests Dr. Seelig, to prevent chronic magnesium lack as a cause of heart, kidney, and nervous disorders.

Measuring Body Magnesium

Emphasizing its importance in mental function, magnesium is the only electrolyte which has a higher level in the brain fluid than in the blood plasma.

Because plasma magnesium levels tend to stay the same due to homeostasis, it is difficult to obtain a meaningful measure of magnesium in the body. Physicians can check for magnesium deficiency by injecting a measured amount into the vein and seeing how much passes out in the urine. A normal person excretes 90% of the test dose of magnesium, while a deficient individual discharges less, retaining more in the body.

I obtain some idea of the level of magnesium and other minerals with the hair analysis. But hair high in magnesium doesn't always mean the body has sufficient amounts. The hair of persons with low blood sugar frequently shows excessive magnesium and calcium levels, apparently due to a derangement in the body's ability to use calcium and magnesium. The explanation may be adrenal-gland exhaustion, a condition often accompanying low blood sugar, as adrenal insufficiency raises magnesium levels.[15] Sugar intake also raises blood magnesium and promotes its excretion, which may help explain the high magnesium levels found in the hair of those with blood-sugar abnormalities.

At times I detect magnesium and/or calcium depletion by tapping the skin over a major nerve, which causes muscle twitching in the area of the nerve's distribution (Chvostek's sign) if deficiency is present.

Obtaining Magnesium

Processing and refining wheat, sugar, and oil strip away most of the magnesium originally present. Treating frozen vegetables with chelating agents lowers their magnesium content; and soaking and boiling food, as in canning and cooking, causes further mineral loss unless the pot liquor is also consumed.

Magnesium sulfate (Epsom salt), the commonly available form of magnesium, is a useful laxative, because it is poorly absorbed and the magnesium draws water into the intestine which softens and lubricates the feces. But where increasing the body's level of magnesium is the goal, I use chelated magnesium (magnesium attached to protein) because it is absorbed well.

Chelated magnesium is helpful in treating childhood hyperactivity, anxiety, depression, and insomnia. Excessive and prolonged magnesium use can cause drowsiness and stupor, signs of magnesium toxicity. One hyperactive "wild" child on whom magnesium had a calming effect became overplacid and sluggish until I stopped the magnesium, restoring her to a normal level of alertness.

Epsom salt *is* useful as a bath salt, providing a relaxing, soothing bath as some magnesium is absorbed through the skin.

Magnesium salts of bicarbonate, carbonate, oxide, and chloride are also available and somewhat effective, though absorbed less well than chelated magnesium. Dolomite and bone meal are inexpensive supplements containing magnesium and calcium, but unless pure, they also carry lead to the body.

Dietary sources of magnesium are whole grains, green vegetables, milk, nuts, and seafoods. Five to six hundred milligrams daily is the optimal dietary allowance, about half the recommended amount of daily calcium. This is the ideal magnesium to calcium ratio, as too little or too much magnesium to calcium in the diet interferes with calcium absorption.

Though originally a good source of magnesium, nearly all milk these days has added calciferol, synthetic vitamin D. Dr. Lewis E. Barnett reports that calciferol binds the magnesium in milk, making it unavailable. Hard water contains magnesium, but if the water is fluoridated, the fluoride bonds with magnesium in the blood, forming insoluble magnesium fluoride—further evidence that tampering with our natural diet is hazardous.

Sodium (Na)

Sodium and potassium are in a state of dynamic balance within the body. The adult body's 92 g of sodium exists primarily outside the body's cells in the body's fluids and blood plasma, while 90% of the body's potassium is found within the cells. The primary function of sodium is to maintain the body's fluid balance and pressure; thus the higher the level of blood sodium, the higher the blood pressure, and vice versa.

We require 4 g of sodium daily, which we easily receive from foods and salt (sodium chloride) added in cooking and at the table. For optimal balance, we should obtain slightly more potassium than sodium in our diet. Yet the average American consumes two to five times as much sodium as potassium. How does this happen? Grains lose up to 80% of their minerals during the refining process, leaving them with a bland taste. The refined food is then laced heavily with sugar and salt to make the food appealing to the palate. Manufacturers add copious quantities of sugar and salt because it sells. Most of us are sugar and salt addicts, craving far more of these substances than is good for us. These addictions often originate in infancy. In most hospitals, the first nourishment the newborn receives is a bottle of sugar water. Round-the-clock sugar water and the infant is on his way to sugar addiction. As for salt, baby food is often laced with it, not for the baby's benefit but to make the product tasty for Mom and Dad.

Salt and Premenstrual "Blues"

In her book *Killer Salt*, Marietta Whittlesley describes how excessive salt (sodium chloride) in her diet caused depression, irritability, and other symptoms of tension which she experienced with menstruation.

Due to the interplay of progesterone and estrogen, female sex hormones, women retain fluids before their periods. Salt draws fluid, and the liberal consumption of sodium results in excessive premenstrual water retention. This excessive fluid presses upon the body tissues, including the brain, resulting in tenseness and depression.

When Whittlesley drastically reduced her salt intake around the time of menstruation, she no longer retained excessive water and was relieved of her crushing depression.

Not only premenstrual depression, but other depressive states as well can be aggravated by excessive salt intake. If you're feeling blue, examine your salt intake. There is ample salt already present in our foods. Take no added salt and you may be rewarded by improvement in your mood. This observation is supported by the finding that sodium levels in the body's cells are increased in states of mental depression.

Salt and High Blood Pressure

Hypertension is often related to excessive sodium intake. Because salt draws water, it raises the fluid pressure inside the blood vessels. A low-salt diet is therefore often effective in reducing blood pressure.

You might think a person with high blood pressure due to excessive sodium would crave potassium and avoid salt; but exactly the opposite appears true. Excessive salt intake creates an addictive craving for more salt. In a comparison study,[16] hypertensives actually chose more salt in their diet than did normal controls; they preferred copious quantities of the substance which was sending them to an early grave.

Obtaining Sodium

It is usually unnecessary to use additional salt, as we obtain ample sodium in our foods. There are a few exceptions. Persons with adrenal insufficiency or severe low blood sugar and sufferers from sunstroke or extreme perspiration may all experience salt deficiency, resulting in lassitude, weariness, or hot-weather fatigue. In such cases, extra salt in the diet is helpful.

Potassium (K)

The adult body contains about 120 g of potassium, 117 g of which is located inside the cells. Potassium is vital for the function of nerve, heart, and muscle cells, especially the latter. A deficiency of potassium causes muscle fatigue. It is also involved with sodium in maintaining the body's balance between acid and base

Potassium Deficiency, Blood Sugar, and Fatigue

Potassium has a direct effect on blood sugar. Potassium deficiency is associated with abnormality in the blood sugar tolerance test; and when potassium is administered, the glucose tolerance test becomes normal.[17] The diabetes which frequently appears from the use of water pills (diuretics) may be due to the loss of body potassium, potassium-deficiency diabetes.[18]

Hypoglycemics often have a low blood pressure and low levels of potassium as well as sodium in hair analyses. These findings may indicate weakened adrenal function, the adrenals becoming exhausted from the frequent need to secrete adrenalin to maintain an adequate blood sugar. The adrenals also produce mineralocorticoids, the hormones which maintain sodium and potassium balance. With adrenal exhaustion, the ability to produce mineralocorticoids is also impaired. Lacking this mineral-retaining hormone, hypoglycemics lose sodium and potassium.

Potassium deficiency may account for the fatigue hypoglycemics experience, since adequate potassium is needed for muscle function and low potassium causes muscles weakness. Potassium deficiency also causes constipation because of poor muscle tone in the intestines. Heart muscle fatigue causes the pulse in hypoglycemics to be weak, slow, and irregular. Muscle cramps while jogging can signify potassium deficiency. Potassium deficiency can result from chronic diarrhea or from the use of "water pills," diuretics commonly prescribed to reduce high blood pressure, if supplemental potassium isn't given. Excessive sodium in the diet encourages potassium loss through the kidneys.

In addition to muscular fatigue, potassium deficiency causes lack of appetite and mental apathy. Potassium toxicity causes similar symptoms.

Obtaining Potassium

While meat eaters tend to receive excessive sodium in relation to potassium in their diet, strict vegetarians receive a high-potassium and low-salt diet. Fresh fruits, vegetables, and whole grains are rich in potassium.

For the mildly potassium-depleted, I suggest four to six helpings daily of fruit juice or vegetable soup. Most salt substitutes have a high potassium chloride content, such as Morton's Lite salt, which is 26% potassium and only 19.5% sodium. This is an inexpensive means of receiving supplemental potassium. Actual potassium supplements are available, but they are expensive and irritating to the stomach. Dried sea water, sea salt, is only 1% potassium and therefore not a good source. Potassium chelates are easy on the stomach and effective, but also expensive. The two I use are Wamel, freeze-dried watermelon from Miller Pharmacal, and Sero 99 K from Seroyal. They help combat the weakness and fatigue associated with low blood sugar until more potassium can be introduced into the diet. We require 3 g of potassium a day.

Sulfur (S)

Brimstone, the ancient name for sulfur, provided fuel for the mythical fires of Hades. Sulfur ignites gunpowder, matchsticks, and possibly human metabolism. Homeopathic physicians use trace dilutions of sulfur to "speed up" run-down fatigued patients.

This heightening of metabolism may account for sulfur's value in removing toxins and poisons. Sulfhydryl groups, sulfur combined with hydrogen, pull toxic metals, such as lead and mercury, out of the body and also protect against x-ray and other ionizing radiation cellular damage.[19]

Sulfur may help psoriasis, a scaly skin condition which usually erupts on the elbows, knees, and behind the belt buckle. It is commonly used in acne skin creams, and hot sulfur baths have been used for centuries to relieve arthritic and rheumatoid pain.

Obtaining Sulfur

Our daily adult requirement is about 850 mg, nearly all of which comes from proteins, which contain on average about 1% sulfur. The body's 245 g of sulfur is present in four of the amino acid building blocks of protein—cystine, cysteine, taurine, and methionine. The first three amino acids can be made by the body, providing sufficient methionine and/or elemental sulfur is present.

Strict vegetarians on low protein diets can become deficient in sulfur unless they eat red peppers and smelly foods, such as garlic (see below), onions, and chives, which supply generous amounts of sulfur. Asparagus also provides simple sulfur compounds, which gives the typical sulfur odor when passed in the urine.

I prescribe these foods, along with egg yolks, an important source of sulfur, when treating toxic metal pollution. I also use supplements of the sulfhydryl-containing amino acids, cystine and methionine.

For those who cannot obtain adequate sulfur in their diet, a druggist will, on a physician's order, fill number 1 capsules with flowers of sulfur. This dose, taken once daily, provides 200 mg of elemental sulfur to supplement what is obtained in the diet.

TABLE 4.

THE BULK MINERALS

Use Only Under a Physician's Supervision

MINERAL	SIGNS OF DEFICIENCY	SIGNS OF TOXICITY	DAILY REQUIREMENT	SUPPLEMENTAL DOSAGE	RICH NATURAL SOURCES
CALCIUM (Ca)	*Extreme:* muscle twitching, cramps, dizziness, numbness, confusion, irritation and spasm of throat, labored breathing, convulsions *Mild:* grouchiness, irritability, tenseness, depression, faulty memory, insomnia, cramping in calves, positive Chvostek's sign, anxiety	Extensive calcification in bones and tissues	Adult—1 g Pregnant/ lactating woman—1.5 g Child—20 mg for every pound	1 g/day for adults as calcium chloride, calcium lactate, or calcium gluconate	MILK, DAIRY PRODUCTS, MOLASSES, VEGETABLES (PEAS, BEANS, CAULIFLOWER, ETC.), BONE MEAL, HARD WATER, DOLOMITE
MAGNESIUM (Mg)	Sensitivity to sounds, twitching, tremors, dizziness, rapid heart beat, aching muscles, fatigue, depression, grouchiness, insomnia, irritability, hyperactivity, anxiety, positive Chvostek's sign	Drowsiness, lethargy, sluggishness, stupor, coma	300–600 mg	400 mg chelated magnesium	WHOLE GRAINS, GREEN VEGETABLES, MILK WITHOUT CALCIFEROL (SYNTHETIC VITAMIN D), NUTS, SEAFOOD
SODIUM (Na)	Lassitude, weariness, hot-weather fatigue, low blood pressure, anorexia, flatulence	Dizziness, swelling, depression, tension, irritability, high blood pressure, premenstrual blues	4 g	Unnecessary, except in adrenal insufficiency, severe hypoglycemia, sunstroke,	TABLE SALT, HAM, PROCESSED CHEESE, BACON, SAUSAGES, DRIED FISH, NUTS, BUTTER

	Deficiency Symptoms	Toxicity	Daily Amount	Supplementation	Food Sources
(SODIUM, continued)				excessive perspiration use added salt (sodium chloride) or salt tablets—10 g per day of sodium or 25 g of salt	
POTASSIUM (K)	Muscle fatigue: constipation; weak, slow, irregular pulse; muscle cramps while jogging; lack of appetite; mental apathy	Lack of appetite, apathy; muscle fatigue	3-5 g	Usually unnecessary. Season with salt substitutes, four to six helpings fruit juice or vegetable soup daily	FRUITS, WHOLE GRAINS, VEGETABLES (FRUIT JUICES, VEGETABLE SOUPS), POTATOES, BANANAS
SULFUR (S)	Possibly sluggishness and fatigue	Irritating to skin and lungs; low toxicity internally	850 mg per day	Usually unnecessary	PROTEINS (MEAT, FISH, LEGUMES, AND NUTS), EGGS, CABBAGE, ASPARAGUS, BRUSSELS SPROUTS, ONIONS, CHIVES, GARLIC

Sulfur and Garlic

The organic sulfur contained in garlic is responsible for not only garlic's smell but also, probably, its medicinal benefits. Garlic lowers serum fats (triglycerides and cholesterol), preventing hardening of the arteries, and also has an antidiabetic action, lowering blood sugar.[20]

An antibacterial agent with a high sulfur content called *allicin* has been isolated from garlic. Naturopathic physicians recommend garlic as a sometimes remedy for the middle-ear infections of young children.

The bulk minerals affect the smooth working of the muscles, bones, and nerves of the body, its enzyme activities, water balance, and the proper secretion of digestive juices, perspiration, and urine. Sodium, potassium, calcium, and magnesium are the important bases of the body fluids, which balance off the body's acids, chlorine (Cl), bicarbonate (HCO_3), etc. Vegetables and fruits, when burned in the body, release predominately base-forming elements—calcium, magnesium, sodium, and potassium. Cereals, meats, and seafoods release acid-forming elements—chlorine, phosphorus, and sulfur. Since the acid-forming bulk elements are available in plentiful amounts in our diet, only sulfur was discussed in this chapter. But optimal health depends on a balance between acid- and base-forming foods. A table of the bulk minerals considered here is shown on pages 120-121.

The Elements:
Part Two—
The Trace Minerals

We contain only minute amounts of the trace minerals. They are present in amounts less than 0.01% of our total body weight. But, like the bulk minerals, they are essential for life and health. The known trace minerals are iron [60 parts per million (ppm) of the human body], fluorine (37 ppm), zinc (33 ppm), rubidium (4.6 ppm), strontium (4.6 ppm), bromine (2.9 ppm), copper (1.2 ppm), boron (0.7 ppm), barium (0.3 ppm), cobalt (0.3 ppm), vanadium (0.3 ppm), iodine (0.2 ppm), manganese (0.2 ppm), selenium (0.2 ppm), molybdenum (0.1 ppm), arsenic (0.1 ppm), and chromium (0.09 ppm).

Many other elements are found in the body in minute amounts, such as lead (1.7 ppm), aluminum (0.9 ppm), cadmium (0.7 ppm), tin (0.2 ppm), mercury (0.19 ppm), gold (0.1 ppm), and lithium (0.04 ppm). These trace minerals have no apparent function in the body and are considered nonessential. If present excessively, some are toxic, as is the case with lead, mercury, cadmium, and aluminum.

I have found that several of these minor minerals have major effects on the mind, especially copper and zinc, so let's begin with them.

Copper

Copper is involved in many mental mechanisms and apparently acts as a brain stimulant. Dr. Carl Pfeiffer has observed that when copper is overabundant in the body, it may induce insomnia, irritability, alienation, anger, depression, and even paranoia. I can confirm his findings.

Adults contain only a pinch of copper, 100 mg; yet it is essential to growth and metabolism. Copper is abundant in our diet; we ingest 2 to 5 mg daily from food, from using copper cookware, and from drinking water that passes through copper plumbing. This amount is ample for all our needs, and it is neither necessary nor usually desirable to take copper supplements.

Copper and the Mind: the Case of Harold

Harold from Santa Rosa was thirteen when his senses first went awry. Odors of chewing gum and perfume annoyed him, he couldn't stand being touched, and he saw sparks flashing in front of his eyes. His mind deteriorated throughout adolescence as he found high school's pressures overwhelming. He felt sick in crowds; people appeared to look at him sharply, viciously; cars seemed to speed by. Short-tempered, angry, and depressed, Harold harbored fantasies of committing mass homicide.

He was nineteen, anxious, and unable to sleep when I first saw him. Perspiring profusely, he exuded a foul body stench. I routinely test both hair and blood copper levels in such cases. Harold's hair copper was an abnormally high 74 ppm; normal is 10 to 45 ppm. His blood copper was also high, 152 mg % (normal is 64 to 143 mg %). His blood zinc was 96 mg %, which is low relative to the copper. Optimally the blood should have ten parts zinc for every nine parts copper. In Harold's case the ratio was 15.2 parts copper to 9.6 parts zinc.

I placed Harold on zinc and manganese, as both displace copper from the body. But a month later, his blood copper was even higher (160 mg %) and his zinc had risen only to 116 mg %. Harold felt even more depressed and angry. The zinc and manganese were pushing copper out of the tissues into the blood in the process of excreting it from the body, thus inducing a temporary rise in psychoactive blood copper and making him sicker.

Realizing I had to reduce Harold's copper burden quickly, I placed him on Cuprimine, a chelating agent which chemically attaches to minerals and drags them out of the body. I didn't want him to lose minerals other than the excessive copper, so he also received a special mineral complex to replace all the other minerals (ZiMn Capsules or Vicon Plus). To avoid removal of these minerals, the mineral complex was taken at midday, while the Cuprimine was taken in the morning and evening.

Two months later, Harold achieved a normal ratio of copper to zinc and simultaneously felt better. He noticed after taking zinc in the evening (it helped him sleep), he awakened in the morning with strong penile erections. For a young man too depressed from excessive copper to "get it up" before, this was good news indeed.

"Zinc makes me feel warm and loving," he reported rapturously. "I can tell now when I eat foods high in copper, because I start feeling terrible and mean."

Stopping the Cuprimine, Harold remained on a maintenance dose of zinc. But a few months later, his blood copper rose again to 160 mgm %, while the zinc fell to 120 mgm %. Harold was feeling bad again. Mystified, we sent a sample of his drinking water for analysis and discovered it was very high in copper! Harold found a water certified low in copper and a few months later his blood zinc/copper ratio came into balance and he felt better than he had in years. Today, Harold remains free of depression, paranoia, and sensory misperception.

During therapy, Harold had fragments of metal removed from his hand. The fragments had lodged there when he was a child and a shotgun shell exploded in his hand, not long before he first became ill. Perhaps the copper-containing shell fragment had contributed to his copper poisoning.

Copper and Disease

Dr. S. A. K. Wilson in 1911[1] described a hereditary disease characterized by a more than sixfold increase of copper content in the liver and brain, causing mental illness, other nervous system disorders, and cirrhosis of the liver. People with Wilson's disease usually died until, in 1948, chelating agents were first employed to remove excess copper. Now victims of the disease also follow a low copper diet and take potassium sulfide with meals to prevent further copper absorption. Patients respond to this treatment with at least partial and sometimes total return to health.

In 1941, German physician L. Heilmeyer[2] reported elevated blood copper in thirty-two of thirty-seven schizophrenics. He also found elevated copper in the blood of manic depressives and epileptics as well as in persons intoxicated wth alcohol. Infectious dsease and cancer were also associated with high levels of copper.

Sudden stress rapidly elevates serum copper and lowers serum zinc.[8] Serum copper is also increased in hyperthyroidism, which can produce a paranoid psychosis similar to what I have seen in patients with copper toxicity.

Estrogens increase serum copper and lower zinc. Women often become irritable or depressed when taking estrogen-containing birth control pills. Premenstrual tension also occurs in susceptible women at the time of the month when estrogen, and therefore serum copper, is higher. I use zinc and vitamin B_6 in treating these high-estrogen conditions.

Though pregnancy greatly increases both estrogen and serum copper, pregnant women rarely become seriously depressed.

Pfeiffer's Brain Bio Center reports high copper and low zinc in patients with high blood pressure. The copper, along with any contributing toxic metal excess, is removed with zinc and vitamin C, resulting in a reduction in blood pressure.

Obtaining Copper

Because copper is abundant in our food, cookware, and water, it is generally neither necessary nor desirable to use a copper supplement.

Zinc

A 155-pound adult contains a quarter of a teaspoon (2.2 g) of zinc. A typical American diet supplies 10 to 15 mg of zinc daily, but we absorb less than a third of this. Zinc is reported deficent in the soil of thirty-two states and is only marginally or inadequately supplied in the modern diet. Needed in all metabolic functions, zinc is part of the structure of insulin and may influence the secretion of several other body hormones. Because of its sedative action on the brain, I measure blood and hair zinc in every nervous patient, and often prescribe zinc supplements.

Zinc and the Mind: The Case of Sally

"My memory is poor, not about distant events but about recent day-to-day things. I'm fifty-five, and I used to be a darned good probation officer, but lately I'm not attentive," confided Sally, her voice crisp and tense.

"The chief will call and say, 'Please do such and such,' and by the time I walk to her office, I've completely forgotten what I was supposed to do," she moaned.

"They think I'm so businesslike because I write everything down, but I do that to cover my bad memory. This memory thing is strange. I'll drive over to the neighboring town, and when I arrive I'll realize I have absolutely no memory of the trip or how I got there! It's getting enormously difficult for me to do intellectual work, although I was Phi Beta Kappa at college. I'm not as sharp as I used to be; my thinking is 'foggy' and I have the craziest imaginings!"

"What do you mean?" I inquired.

"Lately I've felt the chief is out to get me, and I think the other officers are against me. I realize there is no basis for my suspicions, but I just can't help myself."

"When did this trouble first appear?" I asked.

"Umh . . . actually I haven't felt right since I started taking estrogen. I was having change-of-life symptoms—hot flashes, fevers and chills, the usual thing—and my family doctor suggested estrogen. And at first it certainly helped. My menopausal symptoms disappeared, I felt more vigorous, looked younger; in fact, my daughter says I'm beginning to look like one of those African fertility figures."

She did look quite shapely and young for her age.

"Anything else bothering you?" I questioned.

"I've been losing a lot of hair and it breaks easily. My hands and feet are cold all the time. But my main concern is my mind. It seems as if I have an altered state of consciousness, as if I'm on one of those mind-bending drugs the kids are using these days, but I never have anything stronger than Lipton's tea."

I examined her fingernails; there were several white spots, indicating the probable need for zinc.

"How much estrogen are you taking?"

"I have the bottle in my purse here. Let's see—2.5 mg. Since this business about estrogen and breast cancer came out in the papers, I've been worried about it. I was on a lower dose, but after my hysterectomy, the doctor increased it."

"Why did you have a hysterectomy?"

"It was a preventive thing; I've had six kids, and the doctor thought it was a good idea—it's only partial, I still have my ovaries. Oh, one other thing: I don't know why I didn't mention it earlier—I'm tired, *all* the time. I have to drag myself around."

Aside from appendicitis when she was fifteen, Sally had always enjoyed good health. She ate a balanced, nutritious diet and had used vitamin supplements for years in a careful sensible manner.

But the glucose tolerance test indicated Sally had reactive hypoglycemia (low blood sugar); and her *blood copper* was a very high 194 and her *blood zinc* only 99 mcg/dl.

"Estrogen raises blood copper and lowers zinc, which may be why your copper is so high, especially relative to your zinc. Since your symptoms suggest copper toxicity and a proportionate zinc deficiency, I'm prescribing zinc.

"You might feel worse before you feel better," I cautioned, "because the zinc will temporarily drive your copper even higher as it's removed from the body."

Because estrogen "uses up" pyridoxine (B_6), I prescribed vitamin B_6, a high potency B-complex, and a typical hypoglycemia diet high in protein, limited in carbohydrate, and frequent eating.

Ten months after commencing treatment, Sally's copper was markedly better, though still high. She must have been carrying a tremendous toxic burden of copper in her tissues for it to take so many months to bring her copper level to a point approaching normal.

As Sally's zinc deficiency was corrected, her sense of taste returned, and her hair stopped falling out and began growing in strong and dark at the roots. She felt good, and her intellectual powers were restored.

"Something else," Sally told me recently, "I suffered an awful scar from my appendicitis operation. It didn't heal properly. Since I've been on the zinc, that scar has gotten much better and is starting to fade. And when I would get mosquito bites, they wouldn't heal; now they heal right away. But the best thing is the mellowing of my temperament. I can actually sit and enjoy life now, something I could never do before. I was always driven, unable to enjoy the moment. The zinc has changed that, and that's the nicest thing. I just wish I could have found out earlier.

"And when I see these girls on the pill, slightly puffy, edemic, phlegmatic, and depressed, I ask them about it, and it seems it always started when they went on the pill."

I prescribe 50 mg of vitamin B_6 with zinc for women on birth control pills who feel nauseated, bloated, and depressed.

Certain patients exhibit deceptively high blood zinc levels, though they have symptoms suggesting a lack of zinc. These cases respond to vitamin B_6, which allows them to metabolize the zinc, bringing their high blood zinc to normal.

Zinc Deficiency

Dr. A. S. Prasad first described zinc deficiency in humans in 1961.[4] Working with twenty-year-old mentally retarded Egyptian and Iranian male dwarfs who had tiny underdeveloped sex organs, Dr. Prasad prescribed 100 mg of zinc sulfate daily. The dwarfs started to grow and develop normal sexual function. The physician traced their zinc deficiency to their cereal grain diet, consisting largely of unleavened bread. Grains contain phytate, which blocks the absorption of zinc. Leavening bread, raising it with yeast, destroys the phytate, allowing absorption of zinc.

The skin of zinc-deficient people may be dark from excessive pigmentation or show stretch marks (striae) on the hips, thighs, abdomen, breasts, and shoulders. Acne also may signify zinc shortage.[5] Hair and nails grow poorly; the hair splits and breaks easily and the brittle nails may exhibit white spots or be opaquely white. Taking zinc causes these white spots to disappear or grow out. It also strengthens the hair and deepens its color.

Wounds which heal slowly may signify zinc deficiency; zinc salts promote healing of surgical wounds.

Zinc deficency may cause sexual difficulties. Girls may experience delayed menstruation or irregular menstrual cycles, while boys may be impotent and have scanty pubic hair and small, immature sex organs.

Painful, aching joints, so-called growing pains, may plague the zinc-deficient youth. One small for his age eleven-year-old had such painful knees and ankles he was unable to run or play sports. I prescribed zinc and vitamin B_6 and his pains disappeared. He experienced a dramatic growth spurt and soon was able to sign up for Little League.

Diabetics and hypoglycemics often experience the cold hands and feet associated with poor circulation, which may indicate a need for zinc.

A disturbed sense of taste or smell may mean zinc shortage. One hundred milligrams of zinc daily stimulated significant improvement in patients who had lost their sense of taste.[6] Remember Harold who was bothered by odors, and Sally who temporarily lost her sense of taste.

Zinc shortage swells the body's canals; so children suffering middle-ear infections due to swelling and closure of the middle-ear auditory (Eustachian) tubes might possibly be helped with zinc. Similarly (I have used zinc to correct allergic swellings of sinus and nasal passageways.) One of my patients, a singer afflicted with an unfortunate nasal twang, experienced a sudden maturation and deepening of his voice when he began taking zinc.

Zinc is part of the insulin molecule and has been found lacking in the pancreas of diabetics. It is added to injectable insulin to prolong its action.

Zinc deficiency is common in alcoholics and increases their tolerance for booze. When the body contains adequate zinc, it reacts strongly to alcohol. The heavy drinker who can "hold his liquor" doesn't have as much zinc and isn't as healthy as the person who "gets drunk on one beer."

Oily skin, hair loss, lack of appetite, apathy, and lethargy are also signs of zinc deficiency.

Zinc toxicity

Though zinc is the least toxic of the trace elements in humans, single large doses will cause vomiting and diarrhea. Excessive zinc can displace copper from the tissues, temporarily exacerbating phychiatric depression by raising blood copper. After a few months of continued zinc therapy, blood copper returns to normal. Too much zinc in the gut interferes with the absorption of iron.

There has never been a reported death from zinc overdose. A sixteen-year-old Iranian, reading that zinc was good for wound healing, spread 12 g (12,000 mg) of pure elemental zinc mixed with peanut butter on bread and consumed it to hasten recovery from a minor wound. The next morning, he woke with difficulty and fell asleep both at breakfast and at school. His sleepiness gradually increased over the next four days, prompting his admission to the hospital. There, he fell asleep frequently, staggered about dizzily, and wrote in an illegible scrawl. By the sixth day he had completely recovered and suffered no permanent after effects.[7]

Though zinc induces drowsiness, lengthy supplementation is not a good treatmet for chronic insomnia, because it can cause copper- and/or iron-deficiency anemia.

Obtaining Zinc

Healthy people needn't take zinc, provided they avoid processed and frozen foods and alcohol. Up to 80% of the zinc is removed in refining sugar and cereal grains. Frozen vegetables are often treated with chelating agents, which also remove most of the zinc. Alcohol flushes zinc and other minerals out in the urine.

A high protein diet of meat, fish, seeds, and vegetables is rich in zinc. Herring and oysters, liver, mushrooms, wheat germ, onions, maple syrup, and brewer's yeast are especially abundant sources; meats and milk are good; whole grains, nuts and seeds, peas, and carrots are adequate; and fruits and refined foods are poor sources of zinc.

The National Research Council recommends 15 mg of zinc daily, with slightly more for pregnant and breast-feeding women. When treating excessive copper, deficient zinc imbalance, I prescribe 80 to 160 mg of zinc gluconate daily and measure serum zinc and copper every six weeks. This quantity of zinc should be taken only under a physician's supervision.

Iron (Fe)

The body contains approximately 4 g of iron, about the amount in a small shingle nail. Our daily iron need is 10 mg for adult men, 15 to 20 mg for menstruating and pregnant women, and 12 mg for children. Vitamin C, copper, and the amino acids in protein all enhance the absorption of iron, whereas excessive calcium interferes with absorption. Iron blocks the absorption of vitamin E, and therefore the two supplements should be taken hours apart.

Over half the body's iron is present in the red blood cells as a constituent of hemoglobin, the protein which transports oxygen to the body tissues. Iron, the red metal, lends its color to the hemoglobin, giving blood its red color.

Iron Deficiency

Is it difficult for you to think clearly and quickly? Can you remember what you ate for dinner and who last phoned you? Are you able to add numbers in your head, or do you need to write everything down? Do you feel depressed, dizzy, and weak? Do you become short of breath quickly when running?

Examine your fingernails. Are they brittle, lusterless, flattened, or even spoon-shaped? Do they have longitudinal ridges? Can you bend the nails over the tip of your fingers? Are your ankles swollen?

Check yourself in the mirror. Are you losing hair? Are you pale? Are the tips of your ear lobes a normal rosy pink or are they white?

Any of these symptoms may indicate iron-deficiency anemia. Lack of iron leads to insufficient oxygen-carrying hemoglobin. The red blood cells, smaller (microcytic) and paler (hypochromic) than normal, cannot transport adequate oxygen to the body. The oxygen-deprived muscles lead to exhaustion and the oxygen-deprived brain the diminished acuity, forgetfulness, and depression of iron-deficency anemia.

Menstruating women lose 30 to 60 ml (2 to 4 tablespoons) of blood with every menstrual cycle, including 15 to 30 mg of iron, and are especially apt to be iron-deficient. Excessive menstrual bleeding results in iron deficiency, and iron deficiency itself may induce too much menstrual bleeding.[8]

Pregnancy places a further drain on a woman's iron stores, because she must share her iron with the developing embryo. Childbirth also depletes iron because of the blood lost during delivery.

Children also need more iron because they are rapidly increasing their numbers of red blood cells. A U.S. Public Health Survey of 12,000 representative Americans found one in three children had iron-deficiency anemia. Crankiness, inattention, and poor school performance have been attributed to iron lack.[9] Chewing clay (geophagia) or paint flakes (pica) contributes to iron lack in children because the dirt and paint chips contain elements that block iron's absorption.

Iron supplements are abundantly available and widely advertised, but if you're pale as a ghost or have other symptoms of anemia, it's best not to attempt to treat yourself. The lack of many other nutrients, such as vitamins B_6 and B_{12}, folic acid, and copper, may cause anemia. Even when anemia is due to iron deficiency, there is an additional question only a physician can answer. Is the anemia due to bleeding? Anemia in the elderly may mean a bleeding cancer.

Iron Toxicity

Iron deficiency is common but rarely dangerous. Iron excess (siderosis) is infrequent but presents an increasing hazard. Excessive iron storage occurs because of overabundant iron intake or from frequent blood tranfusions. The African Bantu ingest more than 100 mg of iron per day, from eating food cooked in iron pots and drinking alcoholic beverages made in iron drums. Cider and wine are also significant sources of iron in the United States and Europe, containing 2 to 16 mg or more of iron per liter. The alcohol increases the absorption of this iron markedly. Most iron is stored in the liver, but when overabundant it is also found in the pancreas, heart, adrenals, and skin, to which it gives a bronze color. Excessive iron therefore primarily causes liver damage and diabetes, the latter because the pancreas is involved. Overabundant iron can cause scurvy, because iron inactivates vitamin C. The lack of vitamin C leads to destruction of collagen, the body's cement. This creates softening of the bones (osteoporosis), especially in the lower spine, resulting in destruction of the vertebrae.

Obtaining Iron

Meats, especially liver and other organ meats, dark green leafy vegetables, dried fruits, legumes, whole grains, and molasses are rich in iron. The iron in meat and liver is better absorbed than that in eggs and leafy vegetables. Because cereal grains contain phytates which block the absorption of available iron, the iron in whole wheat is significantly less well absorbed than the iron in meats and vegetables. Refining removes most of the iron originally present in grains, and therefore many refined grains are "enriched" by adding iron; but the iron originally present in grain is more than seven times better absorbed than are the iron salts added to refined flour.[10]

The usual adult dosage of commonly prescribed iron sulfate or iron gluconate is one 325-mg tablet three or four times a day. It is best absorbed if taken between meals along with 300 mg of vitamin C. These inorganic iron salts can cause nausea, constipation, or diarrhea. Chelated iron (iron attached to a soybean protein) found in health food stores is more efficiently absorbed, allowing lower dosages (50 mg three times a day) which are better tolerated by the stomach. In the treatment of iron deficiency, iron supplements should be used for six months to achieve maximum effect. Overdoses of iron can cause sudden toxicity and a suspected overdose should be reported immediately to your physician or to a poison control center.

Manganese (Mn)

Adults contain about 37 mg of manganese, over half residing in the bones. We require 4 to 5 mg daily, the amount present in an average diet. Manganese is essential for transmitting impulses between nerves and muscles. Just as I sometimes prescribe magnesium to quiet the nervous system, I occasionally prescribe manganese because of its stimulating effect on the nerves.

Excessive iron in the diet reduces manganese absorption, just as excessive manganese reduces iron absorption. I use manganese along with zinc to remove overabundant copper from the body.

Manganese Deficiency

Manganese deficiency in birds causes bone disease (perosis). Deficiency produced experimentally in mammals results in slowed growth, bone abnormalities, reproductive dysfunction, and nerve disorders.

No clear-cut picture of manganese deficiency has yet been described in humans, but in 1964 Dr. L. G. Kosenko measured the whole-blood manganese of 122 diabetics and found it was only half that of normal controls. Since then, it's been demonstrated that lack of manganese raises blood sugar excessively; and giving manganese reverses this type of diabetes.[12]

Psychiatrist Richard Kunin reported low hair manganese levels in patients with shaking tremors (tardive dyskinesia) from the long-term use of major tranquilizers. Manganese (30 to 60 mg per day) improved fourteen of his fifteen cases.[18] This improvement may have occurred because manganese aids metabolism of the B vitamin choline, which also often corrects this condition.

Manganese Toxicity

Excessive amounts may be inhaled by manganese miners and chemical workers. Early symptoms are poor appetite, apathy, weakness, depression, impotence, disturbed sleep, and, occasionally, temporary insanity and violence. The sufferer shows a type of Parkinsonism, with muscular rigidity and tremor, a monotone voice, and a "frozen" masklike facial expression.

Obtaining Manganese

Leafy vegetables, peas, beans, whole grains, nuts, coffee, and especially tea are good food sources of manganese. Manganese is largely lost in food processing. Corn germ, for example, contains 10 mg % manganese, while whole corn contains 1 mg % and commercial corn flakes only 0.04 mg %.

Chromium (Cr)

There are only 20 parts per billion of chromium in the blood; yet this minuscule amount is indispensable to healthy sugar and fat metabolism. Without chromium, insulin is ineffective, causing diabetes; and cholesterol cannot be metabolized, resulting in hardening of the arteries.

Dr. Henry Schroeder compared chromium-fed rats with a control group on a low chromium diet. The rats given chromium grew faster and survived longer. They had normal blood sugars, low blood cholesterol levels, and did not develop atherosclerotic plaques in their aortas, the main artery of the body. The low-chromium group had elevated blood sugar and blood cholesterol levels, and 20% exhibited aortic plaques.[14]

Chromium levels are highest at birth. In the Orient, where hardening of the arteries and diabetes are much less common, chromium levels remain adequate throughout life, but in the West a person's level decreases with age. Adult Orientals have five times as much chromium in their bodies as adult Americans.

The American diet provides 60% of its calories from refined sugar, refined flour, and fat. Most of the chromium is stripped away in processing. Refining sugar from sugar cane, for example, removes 94% of the chromium.[15] Since chromium is required in sugar metabolism, our high sugar and starch diet further depletes chromium. The high incidence of diabetes and hardening of the arteries thus appears to be closely linked to inadequate chromium intake.

Obtaining Chromium

Tablets made from inorganic chromium salts are poorly absorbed. Only 0.5% of the chromium is actually used. To be well absorbed, chromium must be in an organic, biologically active form. Foods containing biologically active chromium are black pepper, liver, beef, whole wheat bread, beets, beer, and mushrooms.

It is estimated that humans require 2 to 6 mg of organic chromium per day. The richest source is brewer's yeast—two heaping tablespoons of the powder or twelve tablets daily. I prescribe brewer's yeast to nearly every patient for its chromium as well as its many other nutritional benefits. For the 20% of the population which can't tolerate brewer's yeast, biologically active chelated chromium supplements are available at health food stores.

Selenium (Sn)

Selenium in toxic amounts is extremely poisonous; yet traces are essential and may extend the life span. Selenium, like vitamin E, is an antioxidant. In animal experiments, antioxidants prolong life; and selenium appears to increase the effectiveness of vitamin E. Selenium is present in human blood. Human breast milk contains six times more selenium than cow's milk and twice the vitamin E.

Selenium Deficiency and Cancer

Dr. Gerhard N. Schrauzer of the University of California at San Diego reports lower amounts of cancer in areas where the soil is selenium-rich and thus the diet is high in selenium. Breast and ovarian cancer in women, prostate cancer in men, and leukemia, lung cancer, and colon/rectal cancer in both sexes all show a lower incidence in selenium-rich areas. Dr. Schrauzer fed laboratory mice a fish diet, rich in selenium, and found they developed breast cancer less often than mice on a milk and meat diet. When two parts per million of selenium was added to their drinking water, the incidence of tumors in the mice was reduced eightfold.

Selenium is unevenly present in the soil of the states; Ohio has the lowest and my native South Dakota the highest soil selenium content in the nation. Possibly the high selenium explains why South Dakotans enjoy one of the highest longevity rates in the country. We Dakotans, enduring blazing hot summers and terrible winter blizzards, used to joke that it just *seemed* as if we lived longer.

Selenium shortage is a suggested cause of cataracts, because the concentration of selenium in a cataract lens is only one-sixth that present in a normal eye lens.[16]

The toxicity of cadmium, arsenic, silver, mercury, and copper is more pronounced in selenium deficiency. Adequate selenium protects against the toxic effects of these metals.

Selenium Toxicity

Excessive selenium is toxic to grazing animals and probably also to humans. Two thousand micrograms daily approaches the threshold of toxicity; symptoms include loss of hair, nails, and teeth, skin inflammation, lassitude, paralysis, and eventually death. Overabundant selenium appears to increase tooth decay. I certainly developed a mouthful of cavities during my Dakota boyhood. But I was also the consummate consumer of candy and soda pop, even hiding coins under a rock by the candy store so I would never have to do without.

Obtaining Selenium

The proper daily amount of selenium is about 50 to 200 micrograms. As all foods lose selenium in processing (brown rice has fifteen times more than white rice, whole wheat bread twice as much as white bread), selenium deficiency occurs more often than selenium excess.

Good food sources are tuna, herring, brewer's yeast, wheat germ, bran, broccoli, onions, garlic, liver, eggs, cabbage, and tomatoes. A relatively new source of selenium is Xerox machines, which emit selenium into the air.

Lithium (Li)

The lightest element, lithium never occurs in nature as the pure metal. The designation "lithium" therefore refers both to lithium ions and to lithium salts. The element was discovered in 1818 by J. A. Arfvedson in Sweden, and its name is derived from the Greek word for stone. It is abundant in sugar cane, seaweed, and tobacco; possibly it is tobacco's lithium content which accounts partially for the soothing effect of smoking.

Lithium carbonate, a white powder, is increasingly used today in psychiatry. Lithium was widely employed in the mid-nineteenth century to treat kidney disease, stones, gout, rheumatism, as well as many other disorders. Enthusiasm extended into proprietary medicines and led to the widespread use of bottled curative lithium waters. Many are still on the market, e.g., Vichy, Apollinaris, Perrier, and Lithee, all at one time promoted for their high lithium content.

Widely distributed in nature and inexpensive, lithium carbonate draws water, making it useful in dehumidifiers and air purifiers. It is also an essential component of hydrogen bombs.

Lithium and the Mind

Soranus of Ephesus early in the second century first suggested alkaline waters, high in lithium, to treat mania. But it was the Australian physician John Cade who first successfully treated manic patients with lithium in 1949. Dr. Cade's discovery, made in a small Melbourne hospital, excited little interest.

Unlike tranquilizers, which are patentable drugs with profit potential, lithium, present in nature, could not be patented. As no drug firm could hold a monopoly on lithium, the profit incentive was lacking. Isolated reports of effectiveness, mainly from Mogens Schou in Denmark, kept the treatment alive until a few dedicated researchers finally introduced it into American medical practice in the late sixties.

Today, although accepted by academic psychiatry as the treatment of choice for manic depressive mood swings, lithium use is only slowly spreading. The dosage required to treat manic excitement is large, 900 to 1500 mg per day. The ability to tolerate lithium increases during the manic episode and decreases when manic symptoms subside. Manic patients retain more lithium than normal controls, excreting the excess in the urine upon recovery.[17] Once adequate blood levels are achieved, recovery occurs in one to two weeks.

Patients are usually maintained on lithium indefinitely, as it prevents recurrence of manic episodes. It seems to prevent recurrence of depressive mood swings as well.

Dr. Nathan Kline, respected American researcher, recently suggested lithium as a treatment for depressive paranoia. I also have found lithium helpful in counteracting depressive paranoia in some schizophrenics. Sigmund Freud first noticed this relationship between paranoia and depression. Depressives live in a pessimistic, malevolent world. By developing paranoia, the sufferer provides himself a focus for the anger underlying every depression. He can fix his anger on an object—the persecutor who is making life miserable. With this invented foe, the paranoid no longer has to admit to his anger and is distracted from his overwhelming depression. Lithium can be dramatically successful in relaxing such individuals, whose tendency to grandiosity and receiving "special messages" is, after all, similar to mania.

Lithium Toxicity

The blood level at which lithium is therapeutic is close to the level at which it is toxic. Therefore, blood lithium levels must be obtained frequently when commencing treatment and at regular intervals throughout. Diarrhea, vomiting, drowsiness, muscle weakness, and staggering indicate toxicity, requiring reduction or discontinuance of lithium.

Excreted through the urine, lithium cannot be used when kidney disease is present. In 40% of patients, lithium therapy causes excessive thirst (polydipsia) and in 12% increased urination (polyuria).[18] Because lithium decreases the kidneys' ability to conserve sodium, it is important for patients to take salt (sodium chloride) and fluids liberally. In rare cases, lithium damages the kidneys' ability to concentrate urine, sometimes for many months after treatment is discontinued.[19]

Lithium may depress thyroid function, requiring thyroid replacement therapy. It causes a shaking tremor (tardive dyskinesia), similar to that caused by major tranquilizers, in 5 to 10% of cases.

Because of these possible side effects, I try to wean patients from lithium as soon as the cycle of psychotic excitements appears to have ended. The serious risk of toxicity requires that lithium treatment be carried out by a physician experienced in its use.

Rubidium (Rb)

Like lithium, rubidium is normally present in the body but considered nonessential. It was first used by Botkin in St. Petersburg (Leningrad) in 1887–88. Botkin prescribed rubidium chloride in daily doses of approximately 1.6 g to ten heart patients and serendipitously noticed a decided improvement in the patients' sense of well-being. By the turn of the century, rubidium was employed as an anti-epileptic and a hypnotic as well as used to treat nervous disorders. Externally, it was applied for eye ailments.

In modern times, Meltzer[20] rediscovered rubidium, emphasizing that it had contrasting properties to lithium and might therefore be helpful in treating depression. Dr. Ronald Fieve prescribed a single 1-g dose of rubidium to depressed patients who hadn't responded to anything else.[21] Though lithium leaves the body quickly, rubidium, a much heavier metal, remains active for several weeks. Dr. Fieve reported 45% were improved after two weeks, 70% after four weeks. Considering the severity of these depressions, this result is encouraging and underlines the necessity for more research on rubidium in the treatment of depression.

One gram of rubidium chloride was also found to help depressed schizophrenics; but if the dose was doubled, the schizophrenics' level of anxiety increased.

Possibly rubidium is a specific antidepression mineral, just as lithium is a specific antimania mineral.

We see that minerals have vital effects on our minds and bodies. Even though they are present only in trace amounts, modest variations in concentration can cause major changes. Too little is known about how vitamins affect the mind and body; even less is known about minerals.

The safest and most effective method of obtaining an optimum mineral balance is to eat organically grown mineral-rich food and to drink highly mineralized hard water. Studies of geographical locations indicate the death rate varies with the hardness of water; the harder the water, the lower the death rate. The Hunzas, Himalayan mountain dwellers renowned for their health and longevity, drink hard glacial water, abundant in minerals.

Artificially softened water replaces the calcium and magnesium in water with sodium. Soft water makes great soap suds, but it's not great for our bodies. If you have a water softener, connect it only to the hot water tap, or else drink bottled spring water.

Where bottled waters are concerned, I prefer natural spring waters to distilled water. Distilling water removes the minerals. Some authorities tout it because it reduces the possibility of an overabundance of minerals. But today when many foods are mineral-deficient because of the soil they were grown on or the processing or cooking methods used, we need more than ever a mineral-rich, hard drinking water.

Following is a table of the trace elements discussed. The next chapter considers the toxic metals.

TABLE 5

THE TRACE MINERALS

Use Only Under Physician's Guidance

MINERAL	POSSIBLE SIGNS OF DEFICIENCY	POSSIBLE SIGNS OF TOXICITY	DAILY REQUIREMENT	SUPPLEMENTAL DOSAGE	RICH NATURAL SOURCES
COPPER (Cu)	Anemia with weakness, labored breathing, skin sores	Brain stimulation, insomnia, "racing mind," irritability, alienation, anger, paranoia, aggressiveness, depression, hyperactivity in children, autism, stuttering, brittle hair, premenstrual tension	2 mg	Generally unnecessary	WHOLE RICE, LIVER, CAULIFLOWER, CHOCOLATE, GREEN PEAS, KALE, MOLASSES, MUSHROOMS, GREEN BEANS, PECANS, PEANUTS, WALNUTS, OYSTERS, SOYBEANS, WHEAT GERM, COFFEE, TEA, YEAST, GELATIN, BRAN, SEEDS, LOBSTER, CRAB
ZINC (Zn)	Shortened stature, lethargy, apathy, small sex organs, delayed wound healing, loss of taste and smell, poor appetite, childhood hyperactivity, diabetes, stretch marks on skin, acne, impotence and irregular menses, painful joints ("growing pains"), white spots on fingernails, dark skin pigmentation, frequent infections, hair loss, poor circulation (?)	Vomiting, diarrhea, drowsiness, induces copper- and/or iron-deficiency anemia	15 mg	30 mg daily	MEAT, FISH, SEEDS, WHEAT GERM, ONIONS, MAPLE SYRUP, MUSHROOMS, BREWER'S YEAST, MILK, WHOLE GRAINS, NUTS, PEAS, CARROTS, VEGETABLES, HERRING, OYSTERS, LIVER

Element	Deficiency symptoms	Requirement	Toxicity symptoms	Supplemental dosage	Food sources
IRON (Fe)	Anemia with difficulty in concentration, poor memory, depression, dizziness, weakness, labored breathing, brittle, lusterless, flattened or spoon-shaped nails, swollen ankles, hair loss, pale skin, exhaustion	10 mg adult men 12 mg teenagers 15 to 20 mg for menstruating and pregnant women	Liver toxicity, induced vitamin C deficiency, metallic gray hue to skin or "bronzing" of skin	325 mg of iron sulfate or gluconate 3 to 4 times daily	MEATS, LIVER AND ORGAN MEATS, EGGS, LEAFY GREEN VEGETABLES
MANGANESE (Mn)	Poor bone growth, diabetes, slowed growth of hair and nails, reddening of hair	5 mg	Poor appetite, apathy, depression, weakness, impotence, disturbed sleep, temporary insanity, violence, Parkinsonism (muscular rigidity, tremor, monotone voice, "frozen" masklike face)	For tardive dyskinesia 30 to 60 mg daily	LEAFY VEGETABLES, PEAS, BEANS, WHOLE GRAINS, NUTS, COFFEE AND TEA
CHROMIUM (Cr)	Diabetes?, hardening of the arteries?	Unknown	Unknown	50 to 200 micrograms	BREWER'S YEAST, MUSHROOMS, BLACK PEPPER, LIVER, BEEF, WHOLE WHEAT BREAD, BEETS, BEER
SELENIUM (Sn)	Prevents oxidation, prevents cancer?, prevents cataracts?	50 to 200 micrograms	"Blind staggers" in animals, loss of hair, nails, teeth, skin inflammation, lassitude, paralysis, death	50 micrograms	TUNA, HERRING, BRAN, BREWER'S YEAST, WHEAT GERM, BROCCOLI, EGGS, ONIONS, GARLIC, LIVER, CABBAGE, TOMATOES
LITHIUM (Li)	Manic-depressive disorder, psychotic excitements	No known requirement	Diarrhea, vomiting, drowsiness, muscle weakness, staggering, tremor	900 to 1500 mg only with physician's prescription	TOBACCO, SUGAR CANE, SEAWEED, MINERAL WATERS SUCH AS VICHY, APOLLINAIRE, PERRIER, LITHEE
RUBIDIUM (Rb)	Depression?	No known requirement	?	1 g—only currently available from a physician doing research	SOYBEANS (160 to 225 ppm), MEAT MUSCLE (140 ppm), MILK (0.57 to 3.39 ppm), VEGETABLES (35 ppm)

Detecting and Avoiding the Toxic Metals

Toxic metal poisoning affects the nerves and brain before other organs of the body, just as nutritional deficiencies do. Our industrial age has removed vast amounts of toxic metals from beneath the earth and spread them through the atmosphere, dumped them in our rivers and oceans, and contaminated our foods as never before in history. Simultaneously, modern food processing has removed many of the nutrients which serve to protect us from these toxic metals.

In rapid succession, we are experiencing epidemic increases in violent crime, hyperactivity and learning disorders in children, mental illness, and cancer. Is there a connection? Obviously there is; the real question is why it has taken us so long to recognize it.

Modern technology need not be a villain. We need not halt "progress" in order to save our lives and our sanity. Technology contains within it the seeds for our survival. The hair analysis, made possible through atomic absorption spectrophotometry, provides an early warning device for detecting toxic metal pollution. We can benefit from industrialization without its "killing" us, provided we are aware of the very real dangers it presents and take steps to control them.

Lead

Arthur, a straight-A student, suddenly suffered a severe depression. Severe depression is the usual symptom of chronic lead poisoning in adults. Unable to concentrate, and experiencing strange hallucinations and paranoid thoughts, he dropped out of college.

Arthur came to see me and I ordered a hair analysis, a simple inexpensive procedure which cost him $20 and two tablespoons of hair. His hair lead was very high, 160 ppm. Arthur lived next to a freeway which emitted excessive airborne lead. Like many urban college students, he had been feeding his fine mind a diet of "fast foods" and cola drinks. Such refined foods are deficient in the normal minerals. A body depleted in these normal minerals is more likely to absorb toxic metal pollutants.

Treatment included 6 g of vitamin C daily. Vitamin C helps pull lead as well as other toxic metals out of the body. Arthur was prescribed the amino acids cystine and methionine and advised to eat eggs and baked beans frequently because they provide lead-removing sulfhydryl groups. He was also given generous supplements of the normal minerals.

Two months later, Arthur felt well enough to return to school. Soon he stopped taking his supplements. Not long after, Arthur's symptoms returned and he dropped out of school again. After lead is initially removed from metabolically active tissues, lead stored in the bones is flushed out and enters the blood and brain tissues. This probably accounted for Arthur's renewed symptoms of lead poisoning. These gentle nutritional methods sometimes take as long as two years to clear heavy metal pollutants from the body. When Arthur resumed his lead-recoving regime, his mental symptoms again disappeared and he returned to college.

Symptoms of Lead Poisoning

Headache, excitement, restlessness, agitation, irritability, and especially depression all suggest lead poisoning. Memory and the ability to concentrate are impaired. The sufferer may be plagued with insomnia and nightmares. Hallucinations and other sensory dysperceptions may occur. Muscular aches and pains, nausea, indigestion, and abdominal distress are common.

Sources of Lead Exposure

Primitive humans were exposed to little lead. Analyses of primitive bones have shown no lead content at all. The highest known human exposures to lead, before the age of gasoline, probably occurred in ancient Rome. Syrups and wines were stored in lead goblets. Lead pipes carried water to the houses of the rich. The social scientist S. Colum Gilfillan, in his article "Lead Poison Ruined Rome," offers the theory that lead poisoning resulted in the stillbirths, spontaneous abortions, and sterility which were responsible for the low birth rate of the upper classes of the Roman Empire, leading to the ultimate fall of Rome.[1]

With the advance of Western Civilization have come new sources of lead exposure, the sealant used in tin cans (since 1824, widely since 1865), pewter, candy wrappings, toothpaste, cigarettes (since 1900), insecticides such as lead arsenate (since 1894), paint, bottled wines (since 1800), ceramics and kitchenware glazes, and scores of other elements of modern life.

In 1924, tetra-ethyl lead was first added to gasoline to provide higher octane. Thus was started the most widespread pollution of the human environment by a toxic element that has ever occurred. Today, four million tons of lead are mined and released into the environment every year.[2] Over two pounds of lead per man, woman, and child in this country is burned in gasoline yearly. Half to three-quarters of that comes out of tailpipe exhaust. We absorb 50% of the airborne inhaled lead, amounting to about 38 micrograms daily. This adds to the lead we ingest in our food (300 micrograms), of which only 10% (30 micrograms) is absorbed. We also absorb lead through our skin, fingering newsprint, cleaning engines, working with putty and glazes, etc.[8] It can even enter our systems through the hair as some hair darkening preparations contain large amounts of lead.

Paint is a major source of lead pollution. Lead has a sweet taste, and infants may become poisoned by chewing on painted surfaces (pica). A chip of paint the size of a thumbnail may contain 50 to 100 mg of lead. Old leaded paints contained large quantities, 5 to 40% of the final dried solids. In 1972, the Consumer Products Commission limited the content of lead in interior house paint to 5 mg per gram of paint but has placed no limit on exterior paint. Paint remains a major source of lead pollution.

Even infant food formulas have not been safe from lead pollution. Lamm[4] found that evaporated milk used in commercial infant formulas contained lead because of the lead solder used to seal the tin can. I understand this source of lead pollution has been corrected.

We obtain lead from air, food, and water. Air pollution constitutes our most significant exposure. Residents of remote California mountain areas, breathing cleaner air, have only half the blood lead level (12 micrograms/100 ml) of Los Angeles traffic policemen (21 micrograms/100 ml) and only one-third the level of Cincinnati parking lot attendants (34 micrograms/100 ml). Many studies have shown that urban adults have higher blood levels than rural adults.

We excrete lead. Most ingested lead is excreted unabsorbed in the feces, and most absorbed lead is eliminated in the urine. Skin, hair, nails, and sweat also excrete lead from the body.[5]

Nevertheless, we are not getting rid of body lead as quickly as we accumulate it. Body lead stores increase with age. The body's total lead burden increases from less than 2 mg in children under ten to over 200 mg in persons eighty and over.[6] Most of that lead in adults is stored in the bones. But in children, who absorb lead much more readily (53% of ingested lead is absorbed), the lead is retained in the soft tissues of the body.

North Americans have greater body burdens of lead than do other populations. The Swiss have only 50.7%, the Africans 51.8%, Middle Easterners 64.3%, and Orientals 76.8% the amount present in North Americans.[7]

Lead Poisoning and Hyperactivity in Children

Lead poisoning should be suspected in children suffering with hyperactivity, learning disorders, mental retardation, impulse disorders, autism, and epilepsy of unknown cause.

Dr. Oliver David gave a challenging dose of penicillamine to three groups of children. Penicillamine promotes the excretion of lead in the urine. One group of children were known to be lead-poisoned, the second group were hyperactive children, and the third group normal controls. The excretion of lead was the highest in the first group (325 micrograms per liter). The hyperactive group excreted 146 micrograms per liter, whereas the normal control group excreted only 77.[8]

Dr. David reports that penicillamine therapy also cures childhood hyperactive behavior of unknown cause. Fifty hyperactive children were treated with penicillamine (1000 mg a day in divided doses) for three months. The children with a known cause for hyperactivity were mostly unchanged from the penicillamine therapy; the condition of a few even deteriorated. However, the children with "pure" hyperactivity of unknown cause responded favorably. In every case the hyperactivity totally disappeared, though in some cases there was a short initial period of deterioration. Their average I.Q. score increased from 88 to 97, and their general conduct improved significantly.[9]

A recent study by Dr. Herbert Needleman of Harvard Medical School confirmed that lead pollution lowers I.Q. Dr. Needleman found that the average I.Q. was 4.5 points higher in first and second graders in a white middle-class neighborhood outside Boston who had low lead levels as compared to a group from a similar neighborhood with higher lead levels. Further, 26% of the high-lead children were rated by their teachers as unable to follow a sequence of directions as compared to only 8% in the low-lead category. The children in the high-lead group were much more commonly rated by their teachers as being disorganized, distracted, hyperactive, impulsive, easily frustrated, dependent, not persistent, and having low overall functional ability.

The journal *Chemistry in Britain* notes, "Children and young people appear to be specially liable to suffer more or less permanent brain damage, leading *inter alia* [Latin: among other things] to mental retardation, irritability and bizarre behavior patterns. Lead-induced psychosis is said to show striking similarities to the manic depressive type."[10]

Lead probably interferes with the brain by taking the place of normal minerals like zinc, copper, and iron in the brain's chemical reactions.[11] If the body lacks these normal minerals, it is especially likely to absorb environmental lead. Drinking alcohol enhances the levels of lead in the soft tissues, including the brain.[12]

Blood Lead and Criminal Behavior

At the Full Circle School, Bolinas, California, children come from either Juvenile Hall, other correctional facilities, or the state mental hospital. In general they are urban ghetto children who have grown up in the central city on a "junk food" diet high in sugar and low in minerals. They have received not only lead but also the other toxic metals, especially aluminum, in good measure. When I tested Full Circle children, they showed significantly higher levels of lead and other toxic metals than the general population.

In a study done in Switzerland, blood lead levels averaged twice as high for prisoners (43.5 and 40.5 micrograms per milliliter) as for normal controls (22.4 for blood donors and 21.7 for policemen).[13]

In his new book *Diet, Crime, and Delinquency* (Parker House, 2340 Parker Street, Berkeley, California 94704, $4.95), Alexander Schauss describes a habitual criminal, Tony, discovered to be suffering from lead poisoning. Tony picked up his poisoning by his penchant for oysters and clams, which he ate almost daily. These crustaceans concentrated the heavy-metal pollutants in the water. Tony's clams and oysters came from beaches near a large copper smelter, which emitted lead, along with arsenic, cadmium, and mercury wastes. As a child, he'd absorbed enough lead to affect his learning and behavior. In his early teens, Tony embarked on a ten-year criminal career, the heavy-metal poisoning apparently muddling his judgment.

Not only may lead poisoning cause madness and badness; it may also be shortening our life span. The late Dr. Henry Schroeder of Dartmouth Medical School discovered in an experiment with rats that the addition of 5 ppm of lead to an otherwise lead-free diet reduced the rats' average life span by 24.2%.

Protection from Lead Poisoning

The first rule is to restrict your exposure to lead. Jogging alongside a busy street is an ideal way to increase your lead intake. Joggers should run in uncongested areas, late at night or early in the morning, before the traffic starts.

Live in the country, on the plains, in the mountains, or on the seashore. If you must live in a city, find a hillside where the cleansing winds blow freely. As Maimonides said, "The concern for clean air is the foremost rule in preserving the health of one's body and soul." According to Maimonides, the smoke and pollution of the city, even when it did not cause outright disease, affected the ethereal body of city dwellers; they became duller and morally less sensitive.

Low dietary intake of the normal minerals, such as calcium, magnesium, copper, zinc, etc., increases the toxicity of lead and other toxic metals.[14] Eating refined foods (white bread, white sugar) jeopardizes the body's mineral supplies and allows the lead and other heavy metals present in the body to exert their toxic effect. Further, a body deficient in the normal minerals is more likely to absorb lead and other heavy metals. Consumption of coffee, tea, or alcohol and the use of diuretics promote the loss of minerals through the urine.

Saturating the body with normal minerals protects against pollution from lead or the other heavy metals. A diet high in protein, especially animal protein, provides generous quantities of protective minerals. Organically grown fruits and vegetables are also desirable because of their high mineral content.

Mineral supplements are helpful in avoiding lead toxicity, providing the supplements themselves are not contaminated with heavy metals. Dolomite may be hazardous in this regard, because it is mined in open-pit mines and thus subject to atmospheric lead fallout. Similarly, bone meal, another common mineral supplement, may be contaminated with lead, because lead is stored in the bones of the animals from which bone meal is manufactured. Dr. Richard Kunin describes a Los Angeles woman suffering from lead poisoning who was taking bone meal daily.[15] The bone meal was discovered to have 128 ppm of lead; two tablespoons of bone meal would give her 4 to 5 mg of lead daily. Brewer's yeast, on the other hand, grown on uncontaminated cultures, provides a useful and inexpensive mineral supplement, as well as being 50% protein and rich in the B-vitamins.

Mercury

In 1953, in Minamata, Japan, the cats began behaving peculiarly. Their eyes glazed and they staggered about and went mad, before slipping into coma and dying. Shortly thereafter, the same thing started happening to the townspeople.

By 1958, sixty people had died of mercury poisoning and thousands had become ill. A plastics factory was dumping waste into Minamata Bay, polluting the fish. The cats and the townspeople, mostly fishermen, ate the fish. The mercury content of the fish in the bay was 5 to 15 ppm, about twenty times higher than normal, but the mercury content of the shellfish was even higher, between 27 and 100 ppm.[16] Five thousand years ago, Moses told the Israelites they could eat fish with fins and scales but must not eat shellfish and "creepy crawly things" because they were "unclean." Shellfish living at the interstices between the sea and the land are scavengers and pick up more pollutants than scaled fish.

Consider the expression "mad as a hatter." Mercuric nitrate was used in the felt-making process, and hat makers would get "hatters' shakes" and "hatters' madness" from handling the mercury-containing felt. They were absorbing the mercury through the skin and by inhalation, as did my dentist patient (see Chapter 1), who inhaled vaporized mercury while working with his high-speed drill.

Symptoms of Mercury Poisoning

Psychological complaints, including fatigue, headache, and forgetfulness, are the earliest symptoms of mercury poisoning. Irritability, depression, insomnia, and antisocial personality changes may occur. These are followed by numbness and tingling of the lips, hands, and feet. Later symptoms include weakness progressing to paralysis, "tunnel" vision, hearing difficulties, speech disorders, loss of memory, incoordination, and psychosis.

Chills, fever, cough, and chest pain occur if the mercury poisoning is due to inhalation of mercury vapor. Nausea, abdominal cramps, and bloody diarrhea follow poisoning from the ingestion of mercury.

Sources of Mercury Pollution

Most of the mercury in the body comes from food and air. Big fish such as tuna and swordfish are potential sources of mercury pollution. Fish become contaminated with mercury discharged into lakes and rivers by chemical and paper companies. Bacteria in the water ingest the mercury discharge, and in turn the bacteria are consumed by algae. Small fish eat the mercury-containing algae and the big fish eat the small fish. At each step along the food chain, the concentration of poisonous methyl mercury increases, because mercury, like other toxic metals, is retained in the bodies of fish (and humans) for months and even years.

Fish are not the only food source of mercury. High levels were found in many partridges and pheasants killed by hunters in Montana. Scientists blame the organic mercury fungicides used throughout the state to treat grains. The Montana State Health Department warned, "If a man consumes a two-pound pheasant having 0.47 parts per million of mercury, this individual has used his recommended intake for approximately three or four months."[17]

Because certain forms of mercury can kill bacteria and fugus, mercury is often used as a bacteriocide and fungicide. At one time seed grains used for animal fodder were coated with methyl mercury fungicides, but these products were removed from the U.S. fodder market after a New Mexico family was poisoned eating a hog that had been fed the mercury-coated grain. Three of the children suffered permanent brain damage. Such mercury-treated grain and seed is still available for distribution outside the United States, although it has caused numerous poisoning throughout the world. Frequently the poison warning on the sack is printed only in English.

Dentists and dental technicians are exposed by handling mercury amalgam fillings. Also the high-speed dentist's drill vaporizes the mercury, causing inhalation exposure.

Mercury compounds are added to cosmetics to destroy microbial contaminants. The FDA is concerned that mercury is able to penetrate the skin when cosmetics are applied and perhaps build up toxic levels in the liver and kidneys.[18]

Aluminum

Joan wasn't feeling well. She was nauseous, bloated, and constipated. She was having difficulty concentrating, felt irritable, and complained that her memory had deteriorated. Joan brought in an article from *Prevention* magazine describing the hazards of aluminum cookware.

"My mom uses aluminum cookware for everything," she said. "Could I be suffering from aluminum poisoning?"

Years ago I had noticed that coffee cooked in an aluminum pot upset my stomach, and I had discarded my aluminum cookware. But I was skeptical that aluminum could cause mental disturbances, since all the authorities said it was "inert." Still, I have learned to listen to patients; their hunches are often correct.

The body stores its highest concentration of aluminum in the lungs, liver, thyroid, and brain. If it was interfering with normal function in these organs, it could be responsible for Joan's symptoms. So I ordered a test for blood aluminum level. It came back a very high 240 mcg/dl; the normal range is 10 to 90 mcg/dl. Joan's suspicion had been correct. Now we had a new problem: how would we rid her body of excessive aluminum? The problem of removing aluminum had never been considered before. I decided to consult with Dr. Carl Pfeiffer, the world-renowned expert on minerals and the mind.

"Since magnesium is next to aluminum in the periodic table of the elements, perhaps magnesium will displace the aluminum," he advised. I prescribed magnesium, and a few months later Joan's blood aluminum had fallen to 120 mcg/dl. It had worked. The magnesium displaced the aluminum. As she continued taking the magnesium, Joan's aluminum level eventually fell to a normal 19 mcg/dl, and her irritability disappeared and her memory and ability to concentrate improved.

At Full Circle School for delinquent boys, we've analyzed hair for aluminum ever since the process became available in mid-1977. Every youth has had a higher-than-average hair aluminum level. These boys come mainly from the inner city's lower socioeconomic classes.[19] Aluminum cookware is cheap and therefore a probable source of exposure. Further, over the years they have drunk copious quantities of soda pop and beer in aluminum cans. Since the hair of many of the boys also shows high levels of lead and copper and generally low levels of vitamins, it would be difficult to single out aluminum as the only cause of their behavior problems. Toxic metals often appear to interact synergistically, so that the combined effect of several heavy metals in the body is greater than the sum of effects of each of the individual heavy metals.[20]

Aluminum and the Mind

Dr. L. Kopeloff[21] reported in 1942 that trace amounts of aluminum applied to the surface of the brain in animals will initiate seizures or fits. Dr. I. Klatzo demonstrated that the injection of aluminum salts into the fluid surrounding the brain results in degenerative changes seen in some types of senile dementia.[22] Other scientists have found that cats injected with aluminum are slow learners at experimental tasks.[23] The level of aluminum in the cats' brains is exactly the same as the high level which has been found in the brains of patients suffering with Alzheimer's disease, one type of senility. Thus aluminum may be a poison involved in human senility.

In mid-adult life, victims of Alzheimer's disease lose their memory for recent events. Patients who die from this disease have brain neurofibrillary tangles, cell degeneration; they also show excessive aluminum and silicon in the brain and cerebrospinal fluid. Neurofibrillary tangles have been associated with aluminum poisoning in many common laboratory animals.[24]

Sources of Aluminum

In addition to aluminum cans and cookware, water may also be a source of aluminum pollution. Millions of pounds of aluminum sulfate are used to purify drinking-water systems every year. Not all of the aluminum is filtered out. High aluminum content in the water of New South Wales in Australia has been linked to congenital malformations of the brain. Aluminum is added to most salt to prevent it from caking. Aluminum foil is used to wrap foods. It is used in antacids, deodorants, and baking powder.

As in the case of the other heavy metals, the best means of protection is simply to avoid these sources. Concerned that excessive aluminum might lead to early senility, I read labels carefully. If aluminum is an ingredient, I don't buy the product. Thus I avoid table salt which has aluminum in it, I wash often but don't use deodorants, and if my stomach is upset, I never take an antacid. Why should I eat aluminum, when a little milk will neutralize my stomach acidity just as well without adding to my aluminum burden?

Since aluminum is even put in toothpaste, I brush my teeth with an aluminum-free tooth powder, salt water or baking soda, substances which work as well, cost less, and don't contain artificial sweeteners. (I use Rumford Baking Powder, because it is aluminum-free. Many baking sodas and baking powders contain aluminum. And no, I don't receive any money from the Rumford Company.) If you have aluminum cookware, replace it with iron.

Cadmium

Cadmium can replace zinc in the body and cause hypertension and heart disease. With age, the body accumulates cadmium in the kidneys. The newborn has only 1 microgram of cadmium at birth, but by age fifty, he or she may have accumulated 30 mg, or 30,000 times more than was present at birth.

Sources of Cadmium Pollution

Cadmium exists in balance with zinc in nature. Sufficient zinc protects against cadmium pollution. Refining food removes more zinc than cadmium, disturbing the protective balance. A diet high in refined foods therefore leads to a buildup of cadmium. Soft drinking waters, as opposed to hard, contain excessive cadmium, as does a widely advertised cola drink. Hard water contains calcium and magnesium bicarbonates which precipitate on metal pipes, laying down a hard protective coating. Soft water, especially if it is acid, leaches out metal from the pipes, the most hazardous of which is cadmium.

It is estimated that two million pounds of cadmium was discharged into the atmosphere in 1968 from melting scrap metal for making steel. Cadmium pollution also comes from the burning of coal and petroleum products. Cigarette smoke contains sizeable amounts of cadmium, most of which is absorbed. One cigarette contains about 1 microgram of cadmium; one pack deposits 2 to 4 micrograms in the smoker's lungs. Seventy percent of the cadmium in tobacco passes into smoke, which is inhaled by the smoker or goes into the air to be inhaled by smoker and nonsmoker alike.

Other Toxic Metals

Bromine

Bromine salts, advertised for the relief of acid indigestion, in modest amounts sedate the brain but when used excessively can cause toxicity. Mild bromine intoxication results in fatigue, weakness, irritability, disturbed sleep, slowing of mental processes, faulty memory, drowsiness, and perhaps confusion. Above-average intoxication causes delirium and stupor, thick speech, fear or depression, hallucinations, and a paranoid schizophrenic-like psychosis.[25]

Bismuth

As the subsalicylate, bismuth is present in a proprietary remedy for stomach upset. While the use of bismuth salts for periods of less than four weeks is not harmful, prolonged excessive use potentially can result in poisoning. Toxic symptoms include mental confusion, memory loss, slurring of speech and clumsiness, with accompanying joint problems and muscle twitches and spasms.

Beryllium

Production of beryllium now averages 150,000 pounds a year and is growing at the rate of 20% per year. This increase is largely because of the metal's value in airplanes and rockets. Strong and yet light in weight, beryllium is also highly heat-resistant, melting only at 2500°F. M.I.T. scientists calculate that a person standing 18 miles from where a beryllium rocket is being fired would receive a dose equivalent to that of a person who worked in a beryllium factory twenty-four hours a day for an entire month. Symptoms of poisoning are shortness of breath, weight loss, cough, and phlegm. An inflammation of the lungs results in scarring of lung tissue and heart damage.

Asbestos

Recent studies have caused increased concern about the health hazards of asbestos. Damage from asbestos may not show up for several years, but even exposure for as little as one month can be harmful, because the inhaled asbestos dust tends to remain in the tissues. Cigarette smoking increases the risk of both lung cancer and the lung disease asbestosis in asbestos-exposed groups.

The Hair Analysis

As we have seen, it is now possible to measure mineral levels in hair, a process which has certain advantages over blood analysis. Hair analysis is painless and relatively inexpensive. The cost of measuring eleven or twelve normal minerals plus the toxic metals (lead, mercury, cadmium, arsenic, aluminum) is about $23 to $35, less than one-tenth the cost of obtaining similar information from the blood. Since hair is not as vital as blood, deficiencies and excesses appear earlier. By the time mineral imbalance shows in the blood, the patient should probably be in the hospital. Hair is easy to handle, doesn't smear all over the way blood does, and can be shipped through the mails. If your hair is in short supply and you can't spare the two tablespoons necessary for the analysis, pubic hair can also be used. At this time pubic hair samples are the exception rather than the rule, so tests are not as well standardized as those for head hair and the results aren't as meaningful.

Though hair analysis is a relatively new technique and not available at every commercial laboratory, several now offer it. Here is a list of some of the hair analysis companies:

Doctor's Data, Inc.
c/o Bio-Medical Data, Inc.
Analytical Laboratory
30 W. 101 Roosevelt Rd.
P.O. Box 397
West Chicago, Ill. 60185

Mineralab, Inc.
P.O. Box 5012
Hayward, Calif. 94540

REMEDCO
Analytical Laboratories
14721 Califa St.
Van Nuys, Calif. 91411

M² Ethicals, Inc.
P.O. Box 922
Naperville, Ill. 60540

Spectro Metal-Mineral Profiles
P.O. Box 5701
San Jose, Calif. 95150

There are problems associated with hair analysis which hamper its usefulness. Before analysis, the hair sample must be washed to remove surface contaminants that might contain the mineral to be measured. A standardized washing procedure has not been agreed on, and results from one hair-analysis laboratory do not always agree with results from another. The various washing methods used affect mineral levels differently; some appear to wash out some of the minerals in the hair along with surface contaminants.

Various cosmetic treatments apparently affect hair analysis. For example, bleached hair offers a special problem because bleaching leaches out trace metals; test results on such hair thus show artificially low mineral values. Zinc is increased more than three times by the use of a permanent waving lotion.[26] Certain formulas used to darken gray hair *do* darken hair, all right, apparently by penetrating it with lead. Analysis of hair treated with these darkening formulas will show extremely high lead levels. Since lead can be absorbed into the body through the hair, these people may look younger on the outside at the cost of poisoning their insides.

The color of hair also affects its mineral content. Grayhaired persons have less zinc than do blondes. Blondes have less zinc than do brunettes. Redheads have more iron, the red metal.

The values of minerals found in the hair do not always compare well with those same minerals found in the blood, but early findings indicate hair mineral levels compare well with those in the bones.

The heavier the mineral, the more reliable its value in the hair analysis. Sodium and potassium, which are quite light elements, are unreliable. Magnesium and calcium, somewhat heavier, are somewhat reliable, and values of the heavy minerals like zinc and copper can be measured reliably. The toxic metals—lead, mercury, cadmium, arsenic, and aluminum—are heavy metals and, therefore, accurately measurable in the hair. It is in measuring these toxic heavy metals that hair analysis has its major immediate value.

In order to reflect the body's current metabolism, hair samples should be collected close to the scalp. Healthy hair grows about a half-inch a month. Therefore, analyzing the ends of long hair would describe the mineral status of several months, even years, back.

A hair analysis should be ordered and interpreted by a physician experienced in nutrition.

Toxic metal pollution has been implicated in adult and childhood disorders, as well as cancer, heart disease, and respiratory illness. In my testimony before the U.S. Senate to the McGovern Committee on Nutrition and Human Needs, I suggested that we need a Nutritional Bill of Rights. We are entitled, along with the pursuit of happiness, to clean air, clean water, and clean food.

Neurosis and Blood Sugar

History of Neurosis

The ancient Greeks considered neurosis a physical illness. Their word, hypochondriasis, described a condition of manifold obscure aches and pains—symptoms they believed were due to disorders of the spleen and of the region below the breastbone, the hypochondrium.

Similarly, hysteria derives from the Greek word for the uterus, *hyster*. The ancients believed manifestations derived from the uterus wandering through the body, producing symptoms at each location.

Until the twentieth century, neurosis was considered an organic, hereditary illness. The American psychiatrist George Miller Beard introduced the concept of neurasthenia—literally, "weakness of the nerves"—in 1869. Beard believed chemical changes in nerve tissue resulted in exhaustion of the nervous system. He felt neurasthenia was hereditary and was the price paid for progress and refinement. The precipitating causes were the pressure of bereavement, business and family cares, childbirth and abortion, sexual excesses, abuse of stimulants and narcotics, and "civilized starvation."[1,2]

S. Weir Mitchell (1828–1914), a pioneer psychiatrist in Philadelphia, introduced a successful regimen for neurasthenia consisting of bed rest, restricted activity, and a high-calorie diet.

In 1894, Sigmund Freud proposed separating from neurasthenia a group of disorders which he termed the Anxiety Neuroses.

Freud believed neurasthenia was caused by sexual frustration. "Neurasthenia arises whenever a less adequate relief takes the place of the adequate one, thus when masturbation or spontaneous emission replaces normal coitus under the most favorable conditions."[3,4]

Freud felt the sexual problem in neurasthenia was of recent origin, whereas that in Anxiety Neurosis was to be found in the patient's infancy.

Because of the work of Freud—and Pavlov in Russia—today most neurosis is thought to stem from psychological conflicts. Beard's belief in a chemical cause has been discarded. Though the concept of sexual problems as the agent of all neurosis is questioned, psychotherapy is the accepted treatment.

I do not dispute the psychological view of neurosis; but I find it inadequate. Neurosis exhibits physical, societal, spiritual, and chemical dimensions as well. I approach neurosis from all these levels, especially the chemical.

Correcting the chemical disorder in neurosis changes the neurotic behavior. Neurosis is a reaction to stress. To refer only to psychological stress is limiting. It belittles the multidimensions of stress. Stress gravely affects body chemistry. We burn nutrients at a ferocious pace under the whiplash of stress. A normal person's energy system may meet the challenge of stress; the neurotic's energy system has crumbled under it.

Correcting the chemical imbalances which exist concurrently with neurosis is often the least expensive, most practical, and quickest way to alleviate the condition. I have found that abnormality in the blood sugar nearly always accompanies neurosis. Treating this imbalance generally provides quick and effective help.

While psychological and sexual conflicts may be important in the creation of neurosis, psychological analysis is not always the most effective means of treating the neurotic.

Blood Sugar Abnormalities

In 1924, Seale Harris first identified the blood sugar abnormalities hyperinsulinism and dysinsulinism.[5] Hyperinsulinism is an abnormally low blood sugar (hypoglycemia) accompanied by physical and/or mental symptoms at the time of the blood sugar dip. Dysinsulinism is the combination of an abnormally high blood sugar (diabetes) followed by an abnormally low blood sugar.

Symptoms of Low Blood Sugar

Hypoglycemia has been called "the great mimic" because its symptoms are so varied and widespread that they may apply to many other diseases. It is nearly always accompanied by tension, nervousness, and fatigue. Headaches, neckaches, and dizziness are usual, and often depression, "fits," and blackout spells as well. It may cause speech difficulties, poor memory, confusion, and slowness of thinking. Nausea is frequently present, and sometimes severe abdominal pain.

There is only one definite physical finding in hypoglycemia: soreness and tenderness when pressure is put on the left upper abdomen, over the pancreas. The pancreas secretes insulin, the hormone which drives blood sugar down. The gland is about six to eight inches long and looks somewhat like a bunch of grapes. If you've eaten sweetbreads, you've eaten calf pancreas.

My Discovery About Blood Sugar Abnormality and Neurosis

In August, 1978, at the World Congress of Biological Psychiatry in Barcelona, I reported my findings in ninety-seven neurotics who had received five- or six-hour glucose tolerance tests. These were all patients I had treated in the past six years. Of these ninety-seven cases, eighty-nine, or 92%, had symptoms of their illness (anxiety, fatigue, depression, etc.) during their glucose tolerance test and had low blood sugar.

This startling correlation leads me to the following conclusions. Not only are the common symptoms of neurosis identical with those of hypoglycemia, but the blood sugar pattern in the two appears to be the same. I do not say that hypoglycemia causes neurosis, just as I would not say neurosis causes low blood sugar. I *do* say that one accompanies the other. Each is an expression of the other, occurring at a different level.

The following two case histories illustrate this connection between neurosis and low blood sugar. There are two types of low blood sugar, reactive and flat curve. The case of Carole is an example of reactive hypoglycemia. Susan is an example of flat-curve hypoglycemia.

Carole, a Case of Anxiety Neurosis

Carole, an attractive young woman from Palo Alto, swayed into the office and revealed in a wispy, hesitant, child-woman voice:

"I've been having some discomfort since college, but on Christmas day last winter as I was driving to join my husband in the mountains it hit me. I felt as if my lungs wouldn't work, as if there were not enough oxygen in my body. I stopped the car, got out, and started running, yawning to get air. I broke into a cold sweat and felt panicky and terribly frightened, as if I were going to die. My heart was racing and felt as if it was in my throat."

At a nearby hospital emergency room, Carole received a shot of Valium and the attack subsided. But she continued to experience episodes of panic with a racing heartbeat. She visited several physicians, but electrocardiogram tracings of her heart were always normal.

"One doctor said it was hyperventilation and advised breathing into a paper bag whenever I got an attack. That helped a little, but I'm still depressed and frightened all the time. I have to take Valium to get to sleep at night," Carole continued, "and I drink some wine."

"How much wine do you drink?" I inquired.

"Four or five glasses every night. Even though they say my heart is O.K., I still feel scared about my health. When I was younger I was quite athletic and now I'm not. I've become very frightened, I worry all the time; I can't go where there are crowds because I get anxious. I feel as if I'm going to suffocate."

Carole was a classic anxious neurotic. She had been receiving psychotherapy off and on for ten years and was in therapy now but consulted me because of a lingering suspicion something was physically wrong, a fear which doctors' testings and reassurance had not allayed.

I ordered a five-hour fasting glucose tolerance test. At our next appointment, before seeing the results, she was asked to describe what had occurred during the test. (See Figure 5.)

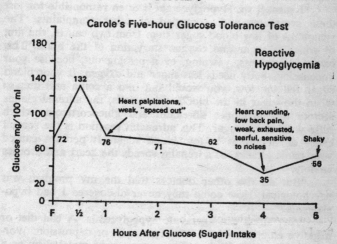

FIGURE 5

Carole's Five-hour Glucose Tolerance Test

Reactive Hypoglycemia

Heart palpitations, weak, "spaced out"

Heart pounding, low back pain, weak, exhausted, tearful, sensitive to noises

Shaky

132

72

76

71

62

35

56

Glucose mg/100 ml

Hours After Glucose (Sugar) Intake

Carole's Reactive Hypoglycemia

"About an hour after they gave me the sugar drink, my heart started pounding and I felt weak and 'spaced out.' By the fourth hour I felt just *awful*. I was very tired, my heart was racing, I got pain in my back, and I started crying."

"During the fourth hour when you felt so bad, your blood sugar dropped to 35 mg %. That's *low blood sugar*," I said.

"And that's what made me feel terrible?"

"Yes. Sugar fuels the brain. It's the *only* form in which your brain can accept food. When your blood sugar falls, your brain cells, starved for sugar, go haywire and you experience mental dis-ease."

"How do I treat low blood sugar? Am I very sick?" she asked anxiously.

"This condition can be completely controlled by changing your diet. People don't die from hypoglycemia, though sometimes it feels as if you will. It's very common and has become more common; 67% of my patients have low blood sugar."

"Is hypoglycemia causing my panic attacks and the heart palpitations?"

"I suspect so. Hypoglycemia is often responsible for just these symptoms and a myriad of other complaints. The symptoms of low blood sugar stem from two causes, the first of which is sugar and oxygen starvation of the brain. This causes drowsiness, yawning, even passing out, because your unconscious body needs less sugar and oxygen. If your blood sugar fell too low, you would fall into a coma and die; so when the sugar in the blood-stream falls, the adrenal glands secrete the hormones adrenalin and glucocorticoid, which raise your blood sugar. This adrenalin reaction is the second cause of symptoms in low blood sugar. It perhaps caused your panic attacks, as adrenalin speeds the heart and arouses anxiety."

"But all the other doctors told me my problem was psychological. How come they never discovered I had hypoglycemia?"

"Any stress can aggravate hypoglycemia. A bad diet or negative emotions—fear, anxiety, anger, or depression. Worrying may put as much stress on your sugar metabolism as a cup of coffee and a hot fudge sundae.

"Psychotherapy, or anything which reduces your psychological stress, may alleviate your hypoglycemia. But immediate help results from adopting a hypoglycemic diet. Exercise also helps. You used to be athletic. Can you resume that? Exercise permits sugar's use in the body's cells without requiring insulin. If you avoid insulin release, you'll also avoid the counterbalancing adrenal hormone response. Sugar or refined starches rapidly enter the bloodstream, causing a sudden elevation in blood sugar. The pancreas reacts to this sudden blood sugar rise by releasing insulin to drive the sugar back down. In your case, insulin over-shoots the mark, driving the sugar too low and causing a roller-coaster ride.

"A diet high in protein and complex carbohydrates such

as whole fruits, vegetables, and legumes is best," I went on, "because these foods take up to five hours to be digested, raise the blood sugar slowly, and don't trigger a massive insulin response. You'll have to give up candy, sugar, pastry, coffee, and wine. And you won't feel better right away; for a time you may feel worse. We are addicted to sugar; the average American eats 125 pounds a year.

"You'll have to avoid the majority of food sold in supermarkets. It may take six months for your system to get back in balance. While others have coffee and donuts, you'll be having cold chicken or carrots and celery. You need to eat every few hours, six or seven times a day."

"I don't want to get fat," she protested.

"You won't. The refined foods you give up are empty calories. When you eat whole unprocessed high-bulk complex carbohydrate and high protein foods, you won't have to consume as many calories to feel full. And you can eat more food without turning it to fat if you have several small meals a day rather than one or two large meals."

When Carole stuck to her high protein diet she did feel better. She stopped drinking wine and fruit juice and her heart palpitations disappeared. Carole began to see clearly the relationship between her mood and what she ate. After a few months of faithful adherence to her diet, one night at a party she indulged in chocolate cake and ice cream and reported the following reaction:

"After eating sugar I felt positively high and very good. Well, I have my sugar problem licked, I thought, but the next day I felt depressed, terrible, and *very tired*. And my face broke out with acne."

When hypoglycemics have been following a diet strictly for a few months, I often encourage them to cheat, as Carole did. Improvement is frequently so gradual that cheating and experiencing the hypoglycemic reaction, which may not be expressed until the next day, helps them recall how miserable they were on sugar and refined starches.

Susan, A Case of Neurasthenia

Susan, from Berkeley, felt apathetic. After ten years of "open marriage," vegetarianism, hot baths, and gurus, she found herself divorced, destitute, and in a state of desultory ennui. Eking out a living giving Swedish massage, she found her infrequent customers, mostly men, usually wanted more than a massage and didn't return when she wouldn't oblige.

In the freedom of their open marriage her husband had "found" himself in a "perfect" relationship with another woman and left Susan because it "just wasn't happening any more." Her ex-husband visited occasionally (his "perfect" relationship petered out after two years), as did a few other men, whenever they were passing through.

Susan smoked a lot of marijuana, didn't eat meat ("bad karma"), and spent a lot of time worrying about her advancing years.

She had a pasty dark complexion with numerous brown "age" spots and poor skin tone. Her voice and general expression were flat, deadpan; her eyes dull, without a trace of enthusiasm. She felt economically, socially, and emotionally trapped.

Susan's Flat-Curve Hypoglycemia

Susan's five-hour fasting glucose tolerance test revealed "flat-curve" hypoglycemia, so called because the blood sugar failed to rise by 50% from the fasting after eating the test meal. In fact it didn't rise at all. (See Figure 6.) This flat blood sugar curve is paralleled by a flat, apathetic emotional state, just as persons with a "hysterical" emotionally labile mood show a widely swinging reactive-type blood sugar response.

Understanding Flat-Curve Hypoglycemia

Drs. Franz Alexander and Sidney A. Portis[6] studied nine neurotics who exhibited flat-curve hypoglycemia, describing them as follows: "The outstanding feature is apathy, a loss of zest, a general let-down feeling of aimlessness, a repulsion against the routine of everyday life, be it occupational activities or household duties. . . . Another constant feature is fatigue, chronic or appearing in acute (sudden) attacks. . . . Along with the more chronic fatigue there may be acute attacks of extreme weakness, tremulousness, sweating and vertigo. At times a feeling of lightheadedness may be manifest. The acute attacks may be associated with anxiety or fainting."

Psychoanalyzing these nine cases, the doctors found the

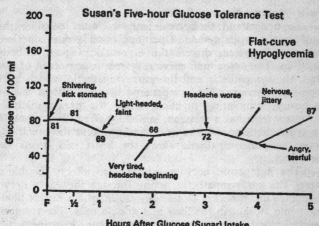

FIGURE 6

Susan's Five-hour Glucose Tolerance Test

Flat-curve
Hypoglycemia

Glucose mg/100 ml

200 — 160 — 120 — 80 — 40 — 0

Shivering, sick stomach

81   81

Light-headed, faint

69

Very tired, headache beginning

66

Headache worse

72

Nervous, jittery

87

Angry, tearful

F   ½   1   2   3   4   5

Hours After Glucose (Sugar) Intake

"outstanding common denominator in the psychological picture of these cases [to be] a lack of spontaneous urge towards the activity in which the patient was then engaged." One man developed his attacks immediately after reluctantly accepting a business position and abandoning his work as an artist, to which he had been deeply devoted. A university student developed her fatigue attacks while forcing her pursuit of career studies. She was torn between her studies and a denied desire for a husband and children. She deeply envied her girlfriends who, one after the other, had married and settled into conventional life. Though she tried to persuade herself she was above such a stupid bourgeois existence, in reality her studies represented nothing but enforced labor to her.

In all cases, the hypoglycemic apathy and fatigue came after the individuals had lost their enthusiasm and zest for life. Their internal protest against feeling oppressed and trapped in a meaningless existence was the flattened blood sugar curve.

Drs. Portis and Alexander treated each of these cases

with a limited-carbohydrate, frequent-feeding hypoglycemic diet, thiamine hydrochloride (vitamin B_1), atropine, phenobarbitol (a sedative), and psychotherapy.

The Autonomic Nervous System

To understand their treatment, we must consider the autonomic nervous system. Operating outside our conscious control, this system directs the automatic vegetative body functions. The autonomic nervous system is composed of two parts, the sympathetic and the parasympathetic, which have opposing functions. The sympathetic nervous system has an excitatory, stimulating function, while the parasympathetic nervous system has a relaxing, inhibitory effect. For example, the sympathetic speeds the heart and quickens the breathing, while the parasympathetic slows the heart and quiets the breathing.

The autonomic nervous system also affects the blood sugar. The parasympathetic, acting through the vagus nerve, stimulates the pancreas to release insulin which moves blood sugar into storage in the liver and muscle cells. The resulting lowered blood sugar causes lethargy, fatigue, drowsiness, and exhaustion. The activating sympathetic nervous system acts through the adrenal gland to secrete adrenalin and noradrenalin. Adrenalin raises blood sugar by pulling stored sugar into the bloodstream, quickening the mental processes, and increasing energy and enthusiasm. Noradrenalin increases our feeling of well-being; it gets us "high."

Drs. Portis and Alexander believed that the autonomic nervous system's regulatory control of blood sugar was out of balance in their neurotic hypoglycemic patients.

Fear and rage markedly stimulate the sympathetic nervous system, endowing humans with super strength to combat the object of the rage or to run away. According to the doctors' theory, enthusiasm and zest for living, striving to achieve heartfelt goals, have a similar tuning-up effect on the sympathetic-adrenal system, less intensive but more prolonged than the stimulation of fear and rage.

It is well known that routine activity, performed without emotional involvement, is more fatiguing even than strenuous activity about which the participant feels enthusiastic.

People trapped in existences they feel are meaningless perform their work perfunctorily, without the zeal necessary to key up the sympathetic nervous system. They unconsciously protest their compulsory activity by creating an emotional state of flight, increasing their desire to give up. Without sufficient counterbalancing sympathetic adrenal tone, the parasympathetic nervous system predominates, resulting in excessive insulin release conducive to relaxation and the storage of sugar. Consequently, those caught in such a situation are unable to raise their blood sugar as is required during activity, causing the low blood sugar symptoms of fatigue, sleepiness, and exhaustion.

A vicious cycle is initiated. The fatigue favors withdrawal, impairing efficiency and discouraging new efforts to continue or resume former activities.

Treatment of Hypoglycemia

Psychotherapy for the flat-curve hypoglycemic is therefore aimed at restoring enthusiasm, thereby increasing sympathetic nervous system tone. Regular physical exercise helps because, as mentioned, it moves blood sugar into the body's cells, providing energy, without requiring insulin. The high protein, limited-carbohydrate, frequent-feeding diet also prevents the strong outpouring of insulin, further reducing the destructive parasympathetic dominance. Drugs, such as alcohol and caffeine, must be avoided because they cause a sudden increase in blood sugar.

Vitamin supplements, expecially of the B vitamins important in energy metabolism, are usually needed. Deficiencies of the B vitamins create fatigue and sluggish energy production. I regularly prescribe the minerals zinc and chromium. Zinc is part of the insulin molecule; and organic chromium (glucose tolerance factor) helps normalize blood sugar.

Blood Sugar and Manic-Depressive Illness

I have noticed that people who experience wide mood swings have similar wide swings in blood sugar. For example, examine Figure 7, the glucose tolerance curve of a thirty-year-old manic-depressive male. Notice that he felt depressed when his blood sugar was as its low.

Many "normal" people feel blue and depressed on awakening. Because they have fasted all night, their blood sugar is low. This mild depression is relieved by the morning meal. People also tend to feel "let down" and experience depressive thoughts in the late afternoon, again when their blood sugar is low. This bleak mood is usually replaced by a good feeling after the evening meal.

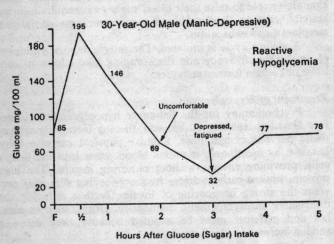

FIGURE 7

30-Year-Old Male (Manic-Depressive)

Reactive Hypoglycemia

(Glucose mg/100 ml vs. Hours After Glucose (Sugar) Intake)

Values: 85, 195, 146, 69 (Uncomfortable), 32 (Depressed, fatigued), 77, 78

Lithium, the mineral which "curbs" the wide oscillations in mood characteristic of manic-depressive illness, also levels out the oscillations in blood sugar levels of manic-depresstives.[7] Perhaps this is one of the reasons it works.

Just as the wide swings in emotional responses of manic-depressives and "hysterical" neurotics are reflected in their widely swinging blood sugar curves, the tendency toward a stoic, unchanging, "apathetic" mood is reflected in a flat blood sugar curve.

Hypoglycemia and Intoxicants

Many hypoglycemics use intoxicants such as marijuana, alcohol, and cocaine to relieve the severe tension they experience. Conversely, hypoglycemia is a nearly universal finding in persons addicted to these substances. Though intoxicants initially raise the blood sugar, causing mental excitation and a feeling of well-being, there follows a reactive fall in blood sugar, aggravating the hypoglycemia.

Marijuana (Cannabis)

Marijuana is now the third biggest business in the country, after General Motors and Exxon. Many hypoglycemics smoke it not only to get high but also to assuage chronic tension, nervousness, and fatigue. Temporarily, it's excellent for those purposes. This is nothing new: the use of marijuana as a painkiller was described by the Chinese physician Hoa-tho in A.D. 200.

The inhalation of marijuana doesn't lower the blood sugar. Actually, there is a slight rise in blood sugar, corresponding to the early excitatory phase of marijuana intoxication. But marijuana causes the "munchies." Why does the body suddenly crave food, especially sweet things, if smoking marijuana doesn't lower the blood sugar? The answer may have been provided by a study of the effects of marijuana inhalation on the liver storage form of sugar, glycogen. Even a single dose of marijuana depleted liver glycogen by half, up to seven days (on the average) after inhalation.

In long-term marijuana users, I commonly see a "paranoid," apathetic, withdrawn state similar to the fatigue state of flat-curve hypoglycemia. I suspect that lengthy use of cannabis aggravates low blood sugar.

Cocaine

Unlike marijuana, which stimulates the appetite and acts as a hypnotic, encouraging sleep, cocaine suppresses the appetite and removes the need to sleep.

While in La Paz, Bolivia, I experienced considerable respiratory distress in the rarefied Andean mountain atmosphere. The least exertion caused labored breathing, and as I yearned to wander through La Paz's exotic but steep streets, I sought a remedy. In the marketplace I purchased a packet of coca leaves, from which cocaine is extracted. The Andean Indians chew coca to stimulate the heart and increase physical stamina, so I decided to follow suit. Chewing the leaves did not induce the mental euphoria associated with using extracted cocaine but nevertheless had a decided effect on my endurance and ability to walk about.

Cocaine is an extremely popular drug. In a recent survey of one hundred drug-using college students,[8] cocaine was *the* recreational drug of choice of all but two of the twenty-nine students who had tried it. In their view, the only limitations on its use were its high cost and lack of availability. If cocaine becomes cheaper and more readily available, dosages will rise and the more dangerous and unsavory aspect of the drug may become more apparent.

Sigmund Freud was an enthusiastic advocate of cocaine's therapeutic potential in his famous 1884 monograph "On Coca": he felt it was useful, among other things, as a treatment for alcohol and morphine addiction. Freud's medical colleague Dr. von Fleischl, addicted to morphine, became the "first morphine addict in Europe to be cured by cocaine." However, von Fleischl, who was using increasing quantities of cocaine by injection, soon became "the first cocaine addict in Europe," and suffered psychologicl disintegration and the paranoid hallucinations of "cocaine psychosis."[9]

In the United States, cocaine was widely used in patent medicines at the turn of the century. Along with many other cola drinks of the period (1886–1903), Coca-Cola used the extract of coca leaves together with other ingredients for flavoring. Coca-Cola was originally advertised as a patent medicine when introduced in 1886—"a valuable Brain tonic and cure for all nervous affections—SICK HEADACHE, NEURALGIA, HYSTERIA, MELANCHOLY, ETC." By 1903, the use of cocaine-containing syrup was abandoned, and instead a flavoring derived from decocainized coca leaves was substituted.[10]

Since cocaine stimulates the adrenal gland, it probably raises blood sugar initially; but as with other stimulants, users report "crashing" depression and fatigue following a cocaine high.

Alcohol

Alcohol, a carbohydrate, acts much like refined sugar and causes a rapid rise and roller-coaster fall in blood sugar. Alcohol mixed with sugared soda is a deadly "double whammy" to the pancreas. Alcoholics unwittingly use alcohol to treat their low blood sugar; their "high" comes largely from the sudden marked elevation of blood sugar. The substitution of tomato or vegetable juice or any food will also raise the blood sugar. Alcoholics who wish to stop drinking should eat high protein food whenever they crave a drink. Large doses of niacin and vitamin C also increase alcoholics' feeling of well-being and help reduce the desire for alcohol.

The Most Common Cause of Low Blood Sugar
—Muscle Tension

Constant chronic muscle tension is experienced throughout the body but primarily in the back of the neck, shoulders, throat, jaw, scalp, and anal sphincter. It is perhaps the most common cause of low blood sugar, as a tense muscle in spasm is a muscle working and therefore burning fuel. Since sugar is the fuel, muscles in spasm cause low blood sugar with its resultant weakness and fatigue.

Here is where the various body therapies fit into a holistic therapy approach. By putting direct pressure on a muscle in spasm, one can break the spasm and induce relaxation, leading to alleviation of the hypoglycemia.

Often "bumps" of tension are located on the back of the head and elsewhere on the scalp. Deep massage of these tension spots will break the spasm of these contracted muscles. When the muscles relax, they lengthen, and the anxious individual will experience relief of the tight, contracted, tense scalp, which may have been causing "bandlike" tension headaches. Similarly, applying finger or thumb pressure under the brow of the forehead helps remove the "worry knot" between the eyes.

The insulin-secreting pancreas is enlarged and in spasm, providing, as mentioned, the only characteristic sign in hypoglycemia: pain when pressure is applied over the left upper quarter of the abdomen, where the pancreas is located. Especially when mental depression is present, the rectus abdominus, the broad covering muscle of the belly, will also be in spasm, and deep massage will provide relaxation. Wilhelm Reich believed that negative emotions lodged in the body and that depression in particular set into the stomach muscles. By holding these powerful emotions, the body tightens into a kind of armor and loses its free flexibility.

Is Hypoglycemia an Allergic Reaction?

Dr. Theron Randolph believes the fall in blood sugar occurring during a glucose tolerance test is an allergic response to the corn sugar used in the glucose test meal. He feels the frequent-feeding, high-protein diet works because it minimizes the intake of the most probable food allergens in their most rapidly absorbed and potent forms. "Those who happen to be susceptible to cereal grains, potato or other foods from which alcoholic beverages are commonly derived, and/or coffee, tea, beet or cane sugar tend to be improved on this dietary program."[11]

Hypoglycemia, Allergy, and Adrenal Exhaustion

Whether low blood sugar is an allergic response to certain foods or allergies are symptoms of hypoglycemia remains unresolved. A person in fragile health and on a poor diet is much more susceptible to any latent allergens. The high protein diet, by strengthening the hypoglycemic's health, protects him against allergies which might have troubled him in his weakened condition. In low blood sugar an endocrine imbalance exists, with a sluggish but ultimately overactive insulin-secreting pancreas and an exhausted adrenal which often functions insufficiently. This adrenal weakness is often experienced as a deep ache in the small of the back.

Adrenal fatigue, accompanying low blood sugar, is not usually detectable by laboratory tests, but general symptoms of mild chronic subclinical adrenal insufficiency usually are present. These include loss of ability to concentrate, lethargy, irritability, depression, weakness, low blood pressure, dark pigmented "age" spots, and low blood sugar itself.

Hypoglycemics often have a general glandular weakness. They have symptoms of poor thyroid function: dry skin, thinning hair, sensitivity to cold weather, slowed mental processes and poor concentration, low body temperature, sluggish metabolism, and weakness. Some show the finely wrinkled pale complexion, and in women failure to menstruate, suggesting an underactive pituitary.

Therefore, gland therapy may help. If adrenal function is sluggish, I prescribe whole adrenal extract tablets with each meal. Whole adrenal gland extract was available for injection and was considered more effective for hypoglycemia than the oral preparation; but the Food and Drug Administration recently removed it from the market. The FDA holds that adrenal cortical extract (ACE) is obsolete because we now have powerful synthetic adrenal hormones. But the synthetic hormones cannot be used to treat low blood sugar because of potent side effects.

When low blood sugar is accompanied by an underactive

thyroid, I prescribe thyroid. Hypothyroidism cannot be corrected if the adrenal is also weak; so I must first make certain that gland is healthy.

Dr. E. W. Abrahamson reports that many asthmatics are aided by thyroid.[12] Asthma, often considered allergic or psychosomatic, is rare in conjunction with diabetes (high blood sugar) but it often occurs together with low blood sugar. Other allergic conditions, including hay fever, occur frequently with hypoglycemia and improve with the hypoglycemic diet. Diet alone doesn't prevent hay fever, but by adding calcium the victim can alleviate such symptoms as the weeping eyes and stuffy nose.

Dr. Abrahamson also found low blood sugar curves in the "psychosomatic" conditions rheumatoid arthritis and stomach ulcers, just as I have found that low blood sugar commonly accompanies neurosis. Perhaps it is the common physical, chemical condition underlying all psychosomatic disease.

10

Allergies and Addictions

One man's meat is another man's poison.
—LUCRETIUS (A.D. 100)

"I learned about the injury food could do to your brain when I was a boy of seven," said ninety-three-year-old Dr. Walter Alvarez at the January, 1978, meeting of the Ortho-molecular Medical Society.

"My mother made the diagnosis. My doctor father didn't make it—he'd never heard that food could affect the brain. But my mother noticed," continued the tall, spare, gnarled patriarch, "that when I ate chicken, I was not myself; I was dulled and often nauseated. And, if I were walking down the street to the post office to get my father's mail, I would lie down on the ground for awhile. My mother said, 'That is due to chicken.' So I quit eating it, and for several years I never had those spells. Then something happened so that I lost this sensitiveness to chicken, and I started eating it again and forgot my former trouble with it. And then I began to have what I called my 'dumb Mondays.' Every Monday, I couldn't write. I could see patients, and I could read, but I couldn't write an article or work on a book. Those were my 'dumb Mondays.'

"I couldn't find the cause until, after a few years, finally

179

I decided it might be food. I kept a record, and sure enough it was chicken on Sunday. My wife always loved to have chicken on Sunday, so I had a dumb Monday.

"Then I had the day when I came out of the mountains with my two sons [Dr. Alvarez, a mountain climber in his youth, credited his longevity to his active physical life], and we hadn't had perfect food in the mountains. . . . We saw a sign, All The Chicken You Can Eat For Fifty Cents. My boy said, 'Dad, let's make 'em lose money!' So we went in, each of us got a small chicken, and we ate it. I was mentally disturbed, headachy, and dull, and I had hallucinations of color and sight. That was a Friday evening that we ate the chicken, and it was the next Wednesday morning before I felt well. That was the worst episode that I ever had.

"Here is another story I think will interest you people who are interested in foods' effect on the brain," Dr. Alvarez continued, "because this was the most remarkable case I ever saw in my whole life.

"In the Mayo Clinic, a young doctor approached me and said, 'Oh, Doctor, I've got a man whose nervous troubles may be due to food; would you mind seeing him?' So I went in, and I immediately whispered to my doctor friend, 'Hey, that fellow's a severe idiot!'

"He replied, 'Yes, I know he's an idiot, but what bothers me is that he wasn't always—he was in the top of his class in the university, and then he changed into this.'

"So I said to the patient's brother, who was with him, 'Was there any other change in his life at the time this happened—when he changed from being a fine student in college to being an idiot?'

"The brother said, 'Yes, our father died, and our grandmother took him into her home. She has a ranch where she raises lots of chickens.'

" 'And what did she feed him?' I asked, my attention alerted because of my own allergy to chicken.

" 'When she discovered he liked eggs, she gave him an omelet of five eggs every morning.'

"And then he had gradually degenerated into this condition. We took him off chicken and eggs of course, and before he left the clinic, he was already much better—said he was going back to college."

Food Allergy Affects All of Us

Food allergy affects nearly all of us, though few recognize that their symptoms are due to it.[1] We don't recognize that our frequent "colds" are really an allergy. We suffer chronic diarrhea, rashes, ringing in the ears, and are completely in the dark as to the cause. We think our headaches or depressions are all due to psychological tensions.

An allergy is a hypersensitive state acquired through exposure to a particular allergen, a substance such as food, pollen, or a chemical to which there exists a specific susceptibility.

Food allergy may express itself as soon as it contacts the gut, causing cold sores in the mouth, nausea, stomach upset, gaseous distension, diarrhea, or constipation with rectal spasm and anal itching; or it may cause symptoms almost anywhere else in the body. Typical hay fever symptoms of watery, itchy eyes, drippy nose and throat, and even labored asthmatic breathing, are common. Fevers, headaches, muscle aches, and skin rashes often occur. Water retention and swelling may signify food allergy, with dark puffy bags under the eyes. Increased water retention from food allergy increases many women's menstrual cramps.

People are most likely to be allergic to milk, wheat, corn, eggs, shellfish, fish, nuts, chocolate, beef, some fruits, and a few vegetables—in short, all the foods commonly eaten. But virtually any food has the potential for causing an allergic reaction.

Food allergy often affects the mind, as did Dr. Alverez' (cerebral) allergy to chicken, causing severe fatigue, "laziness," brain fag, depression (or mania), hallucinations, confusion, migraine headaches, "epileptic attacks," and even psychosis.

Food Addiction is Food Allergy

We are addicted to the very foods to which we are allergic. Just as a heroin addict must continue to "fix" to avoid painful withdrawal symptoms, so a food-allergy sufferer can prevent discomfort only by continuing to consume the addictive substance.

One overweight, depressed young woman addicted to coffee stopped for one week but developed such severe muscle aches, fatigue, and mental depression that she resumed her caffeine.

Characteristically, the allergy-causing substance is a psychic stimulant. It gets the addicted person "high" and therefore makes him reluctant to rid himself of the addiction, even if he knows it is making him sick. When a feeling of well-being is obtained from a substance such as alcohol, cocaine, or chocolate cake, the "high" lasts only as long as the body chemistry is stimulated. As the effects wear off, the person returns to his previous psychic state (not high); and in fact, he will have a compensatory letdown.

One young man had an allergy addiction to wheat. He ate bread and/or cereal every two hours of his waking day. When I first saw him, he was overweight, from both his high carbohydrate diet and his allergic body swelling. He was wheezing, suffering from diarrhea, and mentally depressed. Removal of wheat from his diet cleared up all his symptoms.

One patient had an uncontrollable craving to eat ice cream every night at around nine o'clock. Almost to the second, every twenty-four hours, she would crave ice cream. As if in a hypnotic trance, she would drive to the ice cream store, buy a quart of ice cream, and have a double-dip cone to start on immediately. The rest of the day she was free of craving. Food addiction often has this periodicity.

Food allergy is relative. Quite often, a person may be able to enjoy comfortably, for example, one cup of coffee, but three cups will cause an allergic reaction. Since the food-allergy sufferer is addicted, he won't stop with one cup of coffee; he will drink three or four or ten or twenty cups a day.

Food-allergy sufferers typically have multiple addiction-allergies. They may start their day with coffee and a cigarette, eat sweet rolls for breakfast, and then consume more sugar, coffee, and cigarettes throughout the day. By dinner, they add booze and/or pot, capping it all off with brandy at bedtime.

Psychological Aspects of Food Addiction

Since Pavlov's experiments with dogs, we have known emotions affect digestion. People enjoy better digestion when feeling serene and secure than when feeling anxious or angry.

There is a distinction between hunger and appetite. *Hunger* is a sensation of weakness, signaled by nerve impulses from the gut to the brain and by a dropping blood sugar.

Hunger also means the specific *hunger pangs* felt in the stomach after going without food. Hunger pangs usually last about thirty minutes, then disappear spontaneously for a few hours, but return if a person doesn't eat.

Appetite, on the other hand, is a psychological phenomenon, with a host of causes, and varies widely among individuals, depending on their particular food preferences.

Ideally people should eat only when hungry; but eating is often a matter of appetite, which may in turn be stimulated for a variety of nonnutritive reasons. People eat when feeling *lonely*—the food is something to relate to. They eat because it's *socially acceptable*: at a cocktail party the hostess brings around hors d'oeuvres. They eat when feeling *angry* or *resentful*. Rage leads to the wish to devour and they stuff themselves relentlessly. They eat because something *tastes good*, and they have no will to resist.

Some eat just to *know they've alive;* they are out of contact with their bodies and eat until they can feel their stomachs stretch. Others are *frustrated sexually* and eat to take the place of sex. Eating is often a substitute for *love and security*.

Some eat *in order to be fat;* they want to be "big" people. Others make themselves fat to *avoid sexuality*. Some derive security out of being fat, or they may be trying to incorporate a fat parent into their own psyche. Becoming obese is for them a form of identification.

Many overeat because they have *nothing else to do*. Parents, kept in the house by small children, eat because they can't get away from the kitchen. Along with locking the kitchen as a remedy, they might also junk the T.V., as this passive entertainment, with its frequent commercials for food, encourages overeating.

On the other hand, there are those who are driven to be compulsively thin. In extreme cases, such people lose their appetite completely and may literally waste away and die of starvation, all the while believing themselves to be disgustingly fat. These people are suffering from *anorexia nervosa*.

Two Cases of Compulsive Food Addiction

One patient, a gangly, emaciated academic turned dope dealer, suffered from a form of anorexia nervosa. Though literally skin and bones, he would stand in front of the mirror for hours, bemoaning his "overweight." He did not believe

my assurances that he was not fat. Protein deficiency causes
the belly to swell with fluid, a condition called Kwashiorkor.
This young man had such a protein-deficient swollen abdomen which he was convinced was fat.

Food was for him a compulsive obsession, causing him
to go on eating binges; he gorged on candy, chocolate,
pastries, and ice cream. Immediately afterward, to avoid
gaining weight, he'd race to the bathroom and stick his
fingers down his throat to induce vomiting.

He was pale and gaunt, and his skin was flaking from
nutritional deficiency rashes due to his self-imposed starvation. He had become a recluse, so withdrawn that his girlfriend had left him, a blow which served to worsen his
condition.

Having discovered cocaine's usefulness as an appetite
suppressant, he spent most of his waking hours stoned on
cocaine, marijuana, or Valium.

His tests revealed that he had severe hypoglycemia. I
encouraged him to eat nourishing food and to keep it down.
Informed that his distended belly and emaciated frame were
signs of protein deficiency, he began eating several small high
protein meals a day. He was pleased that protein did not
make him fat but improved his musculature, strengthening his
tentative sense of masculinity. He quickly channeled his
compulsivity into a rigid adherence to his hypoglycemic diet.

Soon he complained that his diet, while healthy, was
boring! I pointed out that he had been seeking sensual
gratification from food. We discussed his frustrated social,
sexual, and career needs, for which food binges had been a
poor substitute.

The self-confidence he gained by mastering his food
compulsion encouraged him to return to school, where he
completed his Ph.D. with honors.

In another case, an attractive but plump young woman
consulted me after a lack of success with crash diets, Weight
Watchers, and Overeaters Anonymous. Her pattern was to
starve until dinner, when she would gorge on French bread,
pastry, cake, cookies, pizza, and ice cream until she sunk into
a somnolent stupor. Her binging left her bloated and depressed, actively contemplating suicide. Her struggle became
so intense that she put a lock on the refrigerator door.

I suggested that if she had to binge, she should binge on
meat, fruit, and vegetables, rather than on ice cream, cookies,

and pastry. Binging on healthy foods did not leave her with as severe a hangover the next morning. Eliminating the allergly-addictive foods from her diet reduced the compulsive craving which accompanied her binges, and her gluttony diminished. Since her binging occurred in the evening, I suggested she go for a walk after dinner rather than stay in her apartment, battling the refrigerator.

Exercise burns calories, provides something to do other than eat, and also moves the blood sugar which the body has accumulated from the evening meal into the body's cells. Not a few fat compulsive eaters have become thin compulsive joggers, turning a negative addiction into a positive one.

She protested she was afraid to walk in her disreputable neighborhood at night. This led to a discussion of her miserable sense of self-worth, which had kept her psychologically trapped in her dissolute area.

Many of her binges had been set off by a man's rejecting her, which was itself inevitable. Lacking any self-respect, she threw herself repeatedly at each new man and clung to him slavishly, addictively. Her pattern illustrates the futility of substituting one appetite for another. Desire is like a flame; the more it's fed, the stronger it grows. The person who tries to substitute unbridled sexuality for compulsive eating usually winds up a fat nymphomaniac! I helped her to see how her indulgence hurt her, and encouraged her to limit her desires.

I applied the principle offered by Hippocrates: "Diseases caused by starvation are cured by feeding up. Diseases caused by exertion are cured by rest; those caused by indolence are cured by exertion. To put it briefly, the physician should treat disease by the principle of opposition to the cause of the disease . . . countering tenseness by relaxation and vice versa."

I countered her self-indulgence by encouraging discipline. Strengthening her self-discipline increased her sense of self-worth. She moved to a safer neighborhood, attended dance and yoga classes in the evening, and as she became slimmer, her natural beauty emerged and she was able to find and maintain relationships with the opposite sex.

This emphasis on self-discipline and will power may seem simplistic. It is reminiscent of the therapeutic technique of Mel Brooks' 2000-year-old psychatrist. He treated a child who, every time she saw paper, tore it into paper dolls. She tore typing paper into paper dolls, she tore menus into paper dolls, and when taken by her distraught parents to see the

2000-year-old psychiatrist, she tore his notepads into paper dolls. How did he treat her? He said, "Little girl, don't tear paper. No, no, little girl, don't tear paper."

The only way to rid oneself of a destructive compulsive addiction is to stop it.

Balancing Addictions

A few greats, such as Benjamin Franklin and Winston Churchill, have successfully managed to balance a plethora of addictions. Churchill was visited by what he termed the "Black dog" in his periodic spells of depression. Churchill, beaten as a youth for stealing sugar, needed feeding at frequent intervals, was dependent on alcohol, and remained a heavy cigar smoker to the end of his ninety years.

The relationship between a depressive nature and great achievement is well illustrated in history, beginning with biblical King David, who would tear his clothes and throw ashes upon himself. Luther, Goethe, and Tolstoy, among many others, were depressives. It may be that these great men fought depression by working obsessively.

Historically, depressives have employed alcohol and drugs; more recently, caffeine, refined carbohydrates, and sugar addictions have been used by depressives to fight their black moods. All such remedies are futile, however, as every stimulant high is inexorably followed by a depressive low.

Detecting a Food Allergy

Many allergists do sublingual, skin, or blood testing in order to discover the food or chemical to which patients are allergic. These tests must be carried out by a skilled physician, and none are completely reliable in diagnosing food allergy.

The soundest test, and one which you can do yourself, is a trial elimination of the suspected food from your diet. Keep a record of everything you eat and drink for one week. Be suspicious of those foods you eat several times a day.

Often a patient remarks he can't be allergic to a certain food because he feels so good after eating it, and objects strenuously to giving it up for testing purposes. Such a food is almost certainly an offending allergen-addictant.

Frequent eating of a food to which one is allergic will not necessarily cause any clear-cut symptoms which allow identification of the offending food allergy, because the sufferer's reactions are masked by continued dosage.

A person may experience fatigue from a wheat allergy but exhibit no clear-cut allergic reaction to wheat because he eats it several times a day. The wheat addict may sniffle in the morning and wake feeling tired and dragged out (because he is beginning withdrawal from the nighttime fast), but these symptoms will be masked by a breakfast containing wheat. Frequent consumption of wheat maintains the addict's partial desensitization. When that person eliminates wheat completely from his diet, he will undergo the aches and pains of withdrawal and then experience a marked improvement. By the fourth day, the person is usually completely recovered. If he then reintroduces a test meal of wheat in his diet, he will experience a full-blown allergic reaction, with diarrhea or stomach cramps, sniffles or sinus attack, possibly skin rash, headaches, depression, nervous tension, or extreme fatigue. The test meal provokes the total unmasked allergic response which was previously obscured by the person's constant use of wheat.

The Pulse Test

Accompanying the allergic response there will usually be a rise in pulse rate by sixteen beats or more per minute, thirty minutes after eating an allergy-inducing food; this provides a simple means of discovering food sensitivity.

The pulse may vary throughout the day, but never by as much as sixteen beats per minute. If the resting pulse varies by more than sixteen beats per minute, it indicates food allergy.

In order to use the pulse test, you must first achieve a basic allergy-free state. To do this with certainty requires a complete fast, drinking only chlorine- and fluoride-free bottled mineral water. Since fasting is difficult and dangerous if not done correctly, you can achieve an allergy-free state by eliminating all the foods you suspect, contenting yourself with a simple diet of lamb, rice, tapioca, and fresh vegetables—foods which rarely cause allergy. Remove shellfish, pork, refined sugar, all cereal grains, and all refined foods. Avoid canned or frozen foods, striving always to eat fresh foods. You must also avoid tobacco, alcohol, and marijuana.

If you have been on such a diet for four to five days, are free of symptoms, and have a stable slow pulse, you are ready to test for those foods to which you may be hypersensitive. Let's assume wheat is one of the foods you eliminated, and you now want to test it. The morning of the sixth day, take your pulse on waking. Let's suppose it's 72 beats per minute. Write down the pulse. Before eating, sitting at the breakfast table, check your pulse again; it's 73 beats per minute. Write that down. Now, having recorded two resting pulses, you're ready to test.

Select a wheat cereal that has only wheat in it—no added ingredients such as sugar, fruit, etc. (hard to find!)—to be certain you're testing your reaction to wheat only. You must eat the cereal dry or washed down with water because you might be allergic to milk and sugar, and you don't want to confuse the results. You need to eat a lot of the test food to obtain a certain allergic reaction, so eat a few bowls; stuff yourself.

Twenty minutes later you feel very good—too good; you're "high," and your heart is pounding. Your pulse is bounding and you clock 102 beats per minute. Obviously you're reacting to the wheat. Your breathing is labored, you've got a sneezy stuffy nose, your eyes are watering, and your stomach feels bloated.

Suddenly, mentally you're no longer feeling high; in fact, you're starting to feel terrible. You're depressed and angry, life looks black and hopeless. Life is a rip-off. Your thinking is negative, and you're developing a migraine headache. *You are experiencing a cerebral-allergic reaction to wheat.*

The violent histamine release set off by the allergic reaction causes swelling of the body tissues, and you look puffy and dark under the eyes.

That afternoon you suffer a violent and sudden diarrhea and take to bed for twenty-four hours. You feel confused and "out of it" for two or three days.

Allergy and the Adrenals

The adrenal gland, the life-preserving gland, is whip-lashed by such dietary stress and substance abuse. Heavy insult exhausts the adrenal strength of all but a few (those with strong hereditary endowment). The consequences of the weakened adrenal function are low blood sugar and the development of allergies. Once this three-way relationship among poor adrenal function, low blood sugar, and allergy is recognized, the treatment of allergy can become the treatment of poor adrenal function. Vitamin C, pantothenic acid, and adrenal-gland tissue may be helpful, as is the removal of adrenal stresses: alcohol, tobacco, marijuana, caffeine, cocaine, amphetamine, and refined sugars and starches.

The importance of healthy adrenal glands in protecting against allergies has been demonstrated by removing adrenal glands from animals. Scientists have determined that the allergic reaction of animals to injection of a foreign substance will be very severe, even fatal, when adrenal glands have been removed, while identical injections affect animals with healthy intact adrenals very little.[2] Sudden allergic reactions are treated with the adrenal hormone cortisone, with excellent temporary success. Cortisone taken internally is not practical in the long-term treatment of allergies because it produces severe side effects.

The stress of an inadequate or overindulgent diet, emotional trauma, infection, insufficient sleep, or the use of alcohol or drugs usually precedes the onset of allergies, with the toxic allergen providing the "straw that breaks the camel's back."

Histamine in Allergies

Food allergies rarely occur when foods are completely digested. Only when digestion is inadequate can undigested or partly digested foods enter the body and, acting as foreign irritants, cause allergies. Most nutrient deficiencies, especially of the B vitamin family, cause poor digestion. When proteins remain undigested, the amino acid histidine, a normal building block of protein, can be converted by putrefactive intestinal bacteria into histamine,[3] the substance which causes the toxic-allergic reaction. Antihistamine drugs are employed to treat allergy but aren't very effective and usually cause drowsiness. Of course, they don't correct the malnutrition which underlies the allergy.

Vitamin C, and the B vitamins pyridoxine and pantothenic acid, all have antihistaminic action and are therefore helpful in allergy. The amino acid methionine (0.5 g, twice daily) and calcium (0.5 g, twice daily) also lower histamine and help allergies.

The B vitamins niacin and folic acid *raise* blood histamine levels and therefore can aggravate allergies. It is probably the release of histamine from the body's mast cells that causes the skin flush in people who take large doses of niacin.

If a person has excessive histamine, this sudden release from niacin may induce panic and a migrainelike headache (histamine headache).

Armoring Your Cells Against Allergens

Healthy cells are enclosed by a membrane which prevents harmful substances from penetrating. A lack of almost any nutrient increases the porosity of this cell membrane, allowing nutrients to leak out and permitting toxic materials to pass in.

Low protein intake, inadequate supply of essential fatty acids, or deficient vitamin E all increase the permeability of the cell membrane. Vitamin A deficiency increases the permeability of cells in the skin and mucous membranes. Vitamin C deficiency also increases this cellular permeability by allowing the membranes' connective tissue to break down. This is how the cold virus penetrates into our cells and brings on a cold. Similarly, foreign proteins can pass through malnourished cell walls, causing allergy.

Taking 5 to 10 g of vitamin C at the first sign of a cold or allergy will "armor" these cell walls and perhaps prevent the onset of the cold or allergy. In the same fashion, protein, essential fatty acids, and vitamins A, B_6, and E in large doses as well as mineral zinc help stave off allergies.

Vitamin C actually fights allergies in four known ways: (1) by increasing the effectiveness of the adrenal gland, (2) by its antihistamine action, (3) by decreasing the permeability of the cell wall, and (4) by detoxifying foreign substances which enter the body.

The vitamin C dosage must be sufficient; 100 mg of vitamin C is not likely to wipe out an advancing allergic reaction, but 10,000 mg probably will. With high doses, I use the sodium form of ascorbic acid to neutralize the acidity. Persons on a sodium-restricted diet cannot use sodium ascorbate but may employ calcium ascorbate.

For the allergy sufferer who does not need to restrict his salt (sodium choloride), sodium ascorbate provides an additional boon. Adrenal weakness which promotes allergies also allows sodium loss through the urine. Since body water follows body salt, when the salt is lost from the bloodstream, it passes into the irritated tissues of the eyes, nasal membranes, intestinal tract, brain (cerebral allergy and allergic headaches), or any affected area and results in allergic swelling. In such cases, one-half teaspoon of table salt or baking soda may provide relief.

Most people are addicted to one thing or another; and food addictions frequently result in food allergy, with its distressing physical and mental symptoms. Often it is not possible to dissipate the compulsive need for an addiction. In such cases the destructive craving can be rechanneled into a positive beneficial addiction, such as exercise, "workaholism," or an exciting hobby, or substituted for with an addiction to largely harmless foods like mineral water, camomile tea, or carrots and celery.

Food addictions can shape and control our day-to-day emotional lives. By knowing and eliminating them, we can escape their enslavement.

11

Sex and Nutrition

The relationship between good nutrition and sex has been known through the ages. Loss of sexual desire and the ability to perform is an early consequence of general malnutrition, as well as a specific symptom of particular vitamin or mineral deficiencies.

Good sexual function requires a healthy body, which in turn requires sound general nutrition, exercise, and sufficient rest. Sexual function in particular is largely controlled by glands, which produce specific chemical secretions. Those glands which secrete outside the body, like the sweat glands, are called *exocrine* glands. Those which secrete internally into the body fluids are termed *endocrine* glands. The secretions from endocrine glands which control our body organs, including our sex organs, are called *hormones*. These glands have specific nutritional needs which must be met to ensure good function and optimal production of hormones. So let's first discuss the glands, their hormone secretions, and their nutritional requirements.

The Pituitary Gland

Located at the base of the brain, this tiny gland is about the size and weight of a pea. It secretes a number of hormones and through intimate connections with the brain (hypothalamus) acts by complex feedback circuitry to influence all the other glands.

The pituitary gland has both direct and indirect effects on the sexual and reproductive functions. The indirect effect is mainly mediated by two hormones, adrenocorticotrophic hormone (ACTH) and growth hormone.

ACTH acts mainly to stimulate the adrenals and is extremely important. Deficiency of ACTH considerably shortens the life span. The B vitamins pantothenic acid and niacin work together with ACTH to stimulate adrenal hormone production.

Growth hormone controls human growth; a deficiency causes dwarfism, while an excess produces a giant.

Gonadotrophic hormones are the pituitary hormones, which have a direct effect on sexuality. In women, they stimulate the development of the egg and the production of female sex hormones. In men, they cause the production of sperm and the male sex hormone. Vitamin E is absolutely necessary to the gonadotrophic hormones' functions.

Vitamin E is more concentrated in the pituitary than in any other part of the body. It is an essential nutrient for hormone production and, acting as an anti-oxidant, protects pituitary and adrenal hormones from destruction by oxygen.

Zinc is also present in high concentrations in the pituitary and affects the secretion of several pituitary hormones. Zinc is key to the function of several other body glands and their secretions; it is abundant in the liver, kidneys, adrenals, prostate, and testis.

Pituitary deficiency is associated with undervelopment of the sex organs. An underfunctioning pituitary causes premature aging, resulting in early menopause in women and impotence in men.

The pituitary depends on complete proteins such as those found in meat, fish, milk, and cheese as well as in whole grains, nuts, and seeds. The B-complex vitamins found in the aforementioned sources and in wheat germ and green vegetables feed the pituitary, especially pantothenic acid, choline, and riboflavin.[1] Brewer's yeast and dessicated liver are excellent B-vitamin supplements.

The Thyroid Gland

Located in front of the throat, the adult thyroid gland is butterfly shaped and weighs up to two-thirds of an ounce (15 to 20 g). Its secretion, the hormone *thyroxine,* controls metabolism.

The thyroid is vital to sexuality. An underactive gland results in lethargy, tiredness, overweight, and lack of desire and capacity for sex. Conversely, an overactive thyroid (hyperthyroidism) races the body's metabolism, sometimes causing psychotic mental excitement and rampant sexuality.

Iodine is the essential constituent of thyroxine; nearly all of the body's iodine (10 mg) is in the thyroid. If one of my patients has a sluggish sex drive and other signs of slowed metabolism, I prescribe 150 micrograms of organic iodine, along with *thiamine* (vitamin B_1), also crucially needed by the thyroid. Normally cold weather and physical exercise spark energy because they increase thyroid function. If they don't, it's a tip-off that thiamine is needed. The other B vitamins and vitamin E are also important.

Certain foods contain an antithyroid factor, goitrin, which depresses thyroid function by interfering with thyroxine's ability to use iodine. These foods are beans, beets, cabbage, carrots, lettuce, peaches, spinach, and strawberries. Iodized salt, kelp (seaweed), and seafood are rich natural sources of iodine.

The Adrenal Glands

Sitting atop the kidneys and pyramidlike in shape are the adrenals, the important survival glands. The combined weight of the pair varies from one-quarter to three-quarters of an ounce 7 to 22 g) as the gland increases in size when stressed. Both physical and psychological stress stimulate the adrenals,[2] but ideally the stress should be positive—for example, encountering a sexually attractive person. The adrenal is composed of an inner core (medulla) and an outer shell (cortex).

The medulla primarily produces *adrenalin* and *noradrenalin*. Adrenalin, the survival hormone, accelerates heart rate and pours sugar into the bloodstream. It raises the blood pressure and directs blood flow to the liver, brain, and muscles; in effect, it makes us super smart and super strong to deal with the sudden stress. It also causes anxiety and inhibits sexual desire. Adrenalin stimulants include the nicotine in tobacco, low blood sugar, exercise, and histamine, as well as psychic or physical trauma. Adrenalin is calorigenic (burns calories), but it's a very nervous way to lose weight.

Noradrenalin, like adrenalin, decreases sexual desire and in the main acts like adrenalin, except that it slows the heart rate and is thought by some to stimulate our feelings of well-being.

The adrenal shell, the cortex, produces three types of hormones: the *glucocorticoids,* such as cortisone, essential for adequate stress response and maintenance of the body's physiology; *mineralocorticoids,* such as aldosterone, which controls mineral balance; and a small but significant amount of *sex hormone.*

Chronic Adrenal Exhaustion

Many persons considered neurotic may actually be suffering from chronic adrenal exhaustion. They complain of fatigue, muscle weakness, loss of the ability to concentrate, irritability, and periods of depression. They have a poor appetite, mild nausea, and usually no strength or desire for sex. They nearly always have low blood sugar, a symptom of adrenal insufficiency. Often their skin is dark, like a suntan that hasn't faded. Or they may have small blotches of brown pigmentation, like freckles. The blood pressure is usually low. Blood sodium tends to be low, blood potassium high; and there is usually a relative increase in the lymphocyte and eosinophil blood cells. Their health is fragile; they may have frequent colds.

If their poor adrenal function is due to diminished pituitary activity, the skin may appear pale rather than darkened.

Such individuals have been on an adrenal "burn out" diet of junk food, high in refined sugar and refined carbohydrate, coffee, and alcohol. Along with prolonged nutritional deficiency, there is often a history of overwork, infections, lack of rest or exercise, and exposure to toxic foods or environmental chemicals preceding the adrenal exhaustion.

Along with regular exercise and a nourishing diet, the specific nutrients I prescribe for adrenal weakness are the vitamins pantothenic acid (250 mg twice daily) and riboflavin (200 mg daily), niacin (100 mg twice daily), vitamin A (10,000 IU fish liver oil daily), vitamin E (200 IU two to three times a day), and most important, vitamin C (3 g daily). Vitamin C is highly concentrated in the adrenals, and adrenal stimulation depletes it. They also requires linoleic acid and the other essential fatty acids, obtained from cold-pressed vegetable oils or wheat-germ oil. I further advise two soft-boiled eggs daily for the biotin and the cholesterol.

Cholesterol is Good for You

Cholesterol has been unfairly maligned by advocates of the low-cholesterol diet. Most of the body's hormones, in particular the sex hormones, are made from cholesterol. It has been demonstrated that high-cholesterol diets, in themselves, don't cause heart disease. The Masai of Tanganyika, for example, live almost exclusively on meat and milk, foods high in cholesterol. They average more than two gallons of milk a day, with 60% of their diet coming from animal fat. Yet their blood cholesterol is low, and they show no evidence of coronary thrombosis or atherosclerosis.[3]

I believe the dietary culprit in heart disease, and in many other diseases, is the use of processed and adulterated foods. Dr. A. M. Cohen reported in 1963 in the *American Heart Journal* that Jews living in Yemen eat high-fat diets but have little heart disease. But when these same Jews migrate to Israel and eat a less primitive, more Western diet, their incidence of heart disease rises to Western levels. Of course, their general exposure to stress also increases with the move to an industrialized society, and stress raises blood cholesterol.

It's true that cholesterol plaques clogging the arteries lead to heart and circulatory disease. But the problem is not cholesterol; the problem is that the cholesterol is not metabolized. A highly processed diet is deficient in the B vitamins, vitamin C, vitamin E, lecithin, magnesium, manganese, and zinc; all of these are needed to metabolize cholesterol. Unable to enter the cells and make hormones, the cholesterol remains in the blood, forming cholesterol plaques. Butter and eggs, then, are perfectly healthy foods, supplying cholesterol and other nutrients needed to make sex hormones for optimal sexual vigor.

The "cholesterol menace" mentality that seeks to replace these vital foods with cholesterol-free food substitutes doesn't solve the real problem; in fact it contributes to it. Two-thirds of American families regularly use margarine, with its chemical additives, in place of butter. Lately, chemical-laden, but cholesterol-free, egg substitutes are being advertised to replace eggs, one of nature's most perfect foods.

Skim milk, in my opinion, is another mistake, as the vitamins and minerals are largely in the fatty portion of the milk. When researchers want to create copper deficiency in laboratory rats, they place them on skim-milk diets. One real solution to high cholesterol is simply to eat less, because blood cholesterol rises directly with increased caloric intake. Increasing exercise and reducing stress also help lower cholesterol. The most sensible diet is one including whole unprocessed foods rich in the nutrients needed to use dietary cholesterol. I prescribe such a diet, high in cholesterol, regularly for my patients, and routinely see a drop in their blood cholesterol on retesting.

The Male Sex Gland, the Testis

Suspended in a sac (scrotum) from the groin, the testis is composed of two glands: the *Leydig cells*, less than 10% of the volume, which secrete the male sex hormone *testosterone;* and the *seminiferous tubules,* 75% of volume, which produce *sperm.*

The adult male produces an average of 7 mg of testosterone daily. Women also secrete a small amount of testosterone (300 micrograms) daily. Testosterone acts to increase sexual desire in both sexes.

Testosterone has therefore been used to treat impotency. But this powerful hormone which also increases aggressiveness can have dangerous side effects, as the following true story illustrates.

"Doc, can you spare a minute?" a patient at a state institution asked.

"Sure, what is it?"

"Can you get me out of here? I'm not crazy and you know it."

"What are you here for?"

"I'm criminally insane—I committed murder."

"Murder, that's pretty stiff; how did it happen?"

"I'm a junkie, right?" he said, flopping into a chair. "I was doing a lot of drugs, living with my ol' lady. She fixed too. I couldn't get it up and my ol' lady sent me to her doctor. He put me on testosterone and it worked pretty good. My wife thought it was great and she started putting the stuff in my food. Man, I had a 'hard on' *all* the time. My ol' lady brought her girlfriends around to enjoy the fun.

"I was using dope (marijuana), acid, (LSD), smack (heroin), Quaaludes, Darvon, and chloral hydrate—and meanwhile taking two or three times as much testosterone as I was supposed to."

I nodded, trying to hide my shock.

"The testosterone made me angry, like a raging bull," he continued without a trace of emotion. "One day I had an argument with my wife in the dime store; then I just pulled out my gun and burned her."

This man used excessive amounts of testosterone, but it shouldn't have been prescribed in the first place. He showed all the sex characteristics of a normal male, indicating his body was producing enough testosterone. Possibly his impotence was due to his heroin addiction, a known cause. Unlike vitamins, which carry minimal risk, hormones can be dangerous and should be employed very carefully.

Testosterone and Marijuana

In a study of twenty young heterosexual males (aged eighteen to twenty-eight) who used marijuana at least four times a week for six months, it was found that their average plasma testosterone was only a little more than half that of a nonmarijuana-smoking control group.[4] The testosterone level was directly related to the amount of marijuana they smoked. Those smoking five to nine joints a week had an average plasma testosterone of 503 nanograms per 100 milliliters (ng %); those smoking ten or more joints averaged only 309 ng % The nonusers had an average plasma testosterone of 742 ng %. Plasma testosterone levels returned to normal within two weeks when users abstained from marijuana.

Since testosterone is correlated with aggression and marijuana often appears to suppress aggressive behavior and increase passivity, lowering of testosterone may be the mechanism whereby this is accomplished.

Sperm

Vitamins A, E, C, and folic acid all work synergistically with testosterone to develop mature sperm and the normal male sex characteristics, such as deepening the voice, developing the beard, male baldness, and enlargement of the prostate gland. Vitamin E deficiency in particular causes degeneration of the testicles and decreased hormone production.

The chemical content of sperm presents certain nutritional implications. The important minerals are calcium (25 mg %), zinc (20 mg %), and magnesium (14 mg %). There is very little copper (0.05%), but sulfur is 3% of the ash. The known vitamin content is vitamin C (13 mg %), B_{12} (300 to 900 ng %), and inositol (53 mg %). Fructose sugar is the main energy source at 224 mg %. Other important nutrients are citric acid (375 mg %), phosphorylcholine (315 mg %), cholesterol (80 mg %), and glutathione (30 mg %). The fishy odor of semen is due to amines such as spermine and spermidine.

Manganese deficiency in male laboratory animals results in loss of sex drive, lack of semen, and degeneration of the seminal tubules. Large stores of the mineral selenium are also present in the testicles and secreted in the seminal tubules. Selenium deficiency has been related to infertility in animal studies.

Zinc is especially important in male sexual function. The prostate and its secretions have the strongest concentrations of zinc in the body. Zinc rides tightly attached to sulfur in the wiggling tale of active sperm. Lack of zinc results in nonmotile, useless sperm.[5]

Dr. Carl C. Pfeiffer reports that the old superstition that excessive masturbation will drive a person insane, or at the very least cause acne, could be true. A good diet provides only 8 to 10 mg of zinc daily, barely enough to prevent deficiency, since only 1 to 2 mg of that are absorbed. A male loses about 1 mg of zinc in the 4.5 ml of ejaculate. A male who ejaculates three or four times a day may therefore develop a zinc deficiency and, as discussed in Chapter 7, zinc deficiency can precipitate acne and even insanity.

Two Cases of Impotence

A young psychologist visited my office complaining of difficulty with erection and shortened staying power. I prescribed two tablets of chelated magnesium twenty minutes before he planned intercourse, which restored and sustained his erection.

Chelated magnesium differs from inorganic magnesium salts in that the electrical charge of the magnesium ion is neutralized by attachment to a protein moiety, allowing much better magnesium absorption.

A middle-aged married stockbroker consulted me because of a lengthy drinking problem, chronic depression, and impotence. His long-suffering wife had decided to leave him, which drove him to me in a desperate attempt to save his marriage. I ordered a complete biochemical workup and again suggested he take two chelated magnesium tablets before attempting sex.

At our next meeting, beaming with restored confidence, he reported instant success with the magnesium. The workup confirmed hypoglycemia, which I'd expected from his history of chronic drinking and depression. He followed a corrective diet, and his depression gradually lifted. When he understood he was drinking as a quick means of raising his blood sugar, he was able to substitute tomato juice for Bloody Marys with obvious benefit.

How do I explain these prompt impotency cures with chelated magnesium? Possibly the power of suggestion, but rational biochemical explanations exist. Alcohol, because of its diuretic action, causes a magnesium deficiency. Refining foods removes much of the magnesium. Our Western diet is high in protein, calcium, and vitamin D, all of which further increase our magnesium need. Depression destroys libido; both of the men I treated were depressed. Total body magnesium is significantly lowered during states of depression and increases after recovery. Magnesium, in chelated form, is often helpful as an antidepressant.

Magnesium is not the only nutrient useful in combating impotence. Dr. Pfeiffer reports that impotence in young men and amenorrhea (lack of menstruation) in young women are most commonly related to a combined deficiency of zinc and vitamin B$_6$ (pyridoxine). The case of Sandra (see Chapter 3) describes this type of disorder in detail.

The Female Sex Gland, the Ovary

Located on each side of the womb are the pair of ovaries, each about the size and shape of an almond. The ovary produces two types of hormones, e*strogens* and *progesterone,* which determine all reproductive functions and shape the woman's sexual features.

The adult menstruating woman produces 0.1 to 0.2 mg of estrogens daily, with a spurt to 0.5 mg on the day the ovary releases an egg (ovulation), which occurs roughly in the middle of the menstrual cycle. Progesterone production is 2.9 mg daily before ovulation and increases markedly to 22 mg after ovulation. Progesterone remains high until the onset of menstruation. Men also produce minute amounts of estrogens and progesterone, mainly formed in the testicles.

Estrogen deficiency in women may result in delayed sexual maturation, with lack of development or shrinkage of the breasts, genitals, and other sex characteristics. Menopause is a normal state of estrogen deficiency.

Deficiency of the B vitamin *folic acid* eliminates the normal response of the reproductive organs to estrogen, resulting in abnormalities in pregnancy. *Niacin* is needed in the synthesis of cholesterol, from which estrogens are made.

Vitamin E is crucial to reproduction and sexual health. Vitamin E is synergistic with testosterone, the hormone which increases sexual desire. The relationship between estrogen and vitamin E is subtle and somewhat contradictory. In some ways, they act antagonistically. Birth control pills, containing estrogen, lower vitamin E levels. Testosterone and progesterone both can be antagonistic to the action of estrogen; and vitamin E works synergistically with both testosterone and progesterone. Yet vitamin E suppositories are used to treat vaginal thinning and inflammation occurring in post menopause women because of estrogen deficiency. *Zinc* also aids in keeping the vaginal tissues healthy.

Progesterone deficiency results in inability to ovulate, interference with menstruation, inability to prepare the womb for the developing embryo, and termination of pregnancy.

Estrogen in Meat

Until the FDA banned it in 1979, 80 to 85% of our livestock were raised on diethylstilbestrol (DES), a synthetic estrogen used to fatten animals quickly, thereby saving on feed costs. Nearly all the increase in weight was due increased animal fat. For the 10% savings in feed bills, meat-eating consumers got fattier meat, laced with hormone residues. Nine other hormones are currently fed to cattle, sheep, and poultry, though some of these hormones have caused cancer in laboratory animals in doses smaller than the amounts present when we eat it at the table.[6] Since meat is our richest source of protein, vitamins, and minerals, it is particularly tragic that this highly desirable food is contaminated with hormones as well as with antibiotics and arsenic.

Until we get our Nutritional Bill of Rights (clean food, clean water, clean air), what should we do about meat? First, since the liver and kidney are the body's filters, where these residues are likely to collect, it is best to avoid eating them. Too bad, since liver and kidney are particularly nourishing organ meats. Dessicated liver tablets are usually made from clean Argentine range-fed cattle and are therefore safe. Plus Products puts this assurance on the label of their dessicated liver.

Second, since these residues—along with herbicides and insecticides used on the grains eaten by livestock—concentrate in the fat, we should follow Moses' biblical admonition and not eat fat. Moses also said we shouldn't eat blood. You can remove much of the fat and blood from meat by immersing your beef or chicken in a large pot of water for half an hour and then let it 'cure' caked with rock salt on a hardboard for a half hour. Afterwards rinse it completely. Water and salt are excellent drawing agents. You will see so much fat and blood in the potful of water, you'll wonder how you ever ate unsoaked and unsalted bloody and fatty meat.

The best thing is to find clean meat. Ask your butcher if his meat is free of chemicals. Tell him that's what you want. Many smaller ranchers and farmers still raise chemical-free livestock. Use the power of the pocketbook; if you demand clean meat, that's what you'll get.

The "Morning After" Pill

Though animals no longer are receiving diethylstilbestrol (DES), many young women still are. DES is the "morning after" pill prescribed to prevent conception after sexual intercourse. This is the same DES prescribed in the forties and fifties to prevent complications during pregnancy. That practice was abruptly ended when it was found that some young women exposed to DES while in the womb, twenty years later developed cancer of the vagina. DES has also been linked to cancer of the womb (uterus) in women who used it during pregnancy.

Birth Control Pills

Despite formidable evidence that birth control pills cause fatal or disabling blood clots, fatal liver disease, cancer, depression, birth defects, and many other problems, they are still widely prescribed.

Dr. Valerie Beral, in analyzing data on British users of birth control pills, found that users and ex-users have a combined risk of death that is higher than that of nonusers. This finding is particularly ominous because women in the pill-using group "were less likely to have a history of previous major illness" than nonusers. The risk of death from vascular disease is three times greater, from suicide four times greater, and from cancer twice as great among users and ex-users of the pill.[7]

A little known fact about the pill is that it changes the acid-alkaline balance of the vagina, increasing the user's susceptibility to venereal disease and other vaginal infections. If a woman has sex with a gonorrhea-infected man, she has a one-third chance of contracting gonorrhea. If she uses a diaphragm with spermicidal jelly, which also kills germs, her chances are much lower. Similarly, foam offers protection against VD, as do condoms. But if a woman is on the pill, her chance of getting gonorrhea jumps to more than 90%.

If you're a young woman who doesn't want to bother with a diaphragm, ask your older sister or friend about her experience with the pill. If you're still determined to take the pill, you should know how it affects your vitamin and mineral balance.

The Pill Causes Vitamin Imbalance

Birth control pills lower body levels of the B vitamins folic acid, pyridoxine (B_6), thiamine (B_1), riboflavin (B_2), and cobalamin (B_{12}), as well as vitamin C and E. Vitamin K may also be involved, and iron and vitamin A levels are increased.[8] Excessive vitamin A is associated with headaches, depression, hair loss, and dry skin. Serum iron levels are elevated because less blood is lost during menstruation if the woman is taking birth control pills, which may be the pill's only good nutritional effect. Birth control pills also raise blood copper and lower zinc. The resulting imbalance may account for the irritability and depression some pills users experience.

Therefore, users of the pill must make a special effort to eat a nourishing diet. They might also use the following suplements: (1) a B-complex supplying 10 mg each of B_6, B_2, and B_1; 0.8 mg of folic acid and 100 micrograms of B_{12}; (2) 200 IU of vitamin E (mixed tocopherols); (3) 1500 mg of vitamin C (this amount corrects deficiency and acidifies body fluids, perhaps helping prevent vaginal infections); and (4) 15 mg of zinc sulfate.

Folic acid, obtained naturally in leafy green vegetables (foliage), may be especially important. One in five pill users develops a suspicious pap smear after three or four years on the pill. Some physicians think this is a precancerous change and recommend surgery. New York City hematologist Dr. John Lindenbaum prescribed pill users with abnormal pap smears 10 mg of folic acid daily by mouth for three weeks, leaving them on the pill. In every case the pap smear returned to normal or near normal.[9]

Menstrual Cramps (Dysmenorrhea)

Many nervous and exhausted young women that I have placed on a high-protein hypoglycemic diet have noticed that their symptoms of menstrual cramping have disappeared. I am not able to attribute this improvement to any particular nutrient; it appears to be a general response to a nourishing diet, with removal of refined sugars and starches.

Women with long, heavy menstrual flow need ample B vitamins, especially B_6 and folic acid. Vitamins C and E, and of course iron, are also required. Since calcium blood levels drop about ten days before menstruation and remain low until the period is nearly over, calcium and magnesium in balanced form often help cramps. Plus Products, Formula 184, four tablets daily, supplies 1 g of calcium and 620 mg of magnesium. I prescribe calcium to be taken between meals with 300 mg of vitamin C and a small amount of fruit juice or milk for maximal absorption.

Aphrodisiacs

Dietary solutions to sexual problems have been sought throughout history. The Book of Genesis mentions mandrake, of the potato family, to increase male sexual desire and potency and to remedy female sterility. Ancient Hindus stressed garlic, onions, leeks, and beans. Contemporary Indian dishes of curry, rice, chutney, mango, and ghee (melted butter) are afforded aphrodisiac value. The *Kama Sutra* most often mentions milk, sugar, honey, ghee, eggs, sesame seeds, wheat, and beans for increasing sexual vigor. The Arabian *Perfumed Garden* similarly praises eggs, milk, honey, almonds, and onions. Chinese aphrodisiacs include onions, bamboo shoots, seafoods, garlic, ginger, and ginseng. Fruits are conspicuously absent from lists of aphrodisiac foods.

Today we understand how some of these foods may

work nutritionally. Milk and seafoods provide high-grade protein, essential for healthy function of the endocrine and sex glands. Egg yolks yield copious quantities of lecithin, needed to produce sex hormones and sperm. Sesame seeds are rich in minerals, vitamins, lecithin, and protein. Honey provides aspartic acid, used by some doctors to treat female "bedroom fatigue." Honey sugars are in a predigested, easily assimilated form, important for the production of male seminal fluid. Oysters, nuts and pumpkin seeds, and red meat all provide zinc, important for the prostate and other sex glands. Butter provides the vitamin A and cholesterol needed for sex-hormone production. Garlic, onions, and leeks are rich sources of sulfur, a metabolic stimulant.

Bird's nest soup, one of the most powerful Chinese aphrodisiacs, is made from the sea swallow nest, prepared out of seaweed glued together with fish eggs. Seaweed (kelp) is an abundant source of minerals, especially iodine, essential for the thyroid. Fish eggs are high in protein, sulfur, vitamin E, and many other nutrients. *Nuoc-man,* a spicy Chinese sauce often recommended as an aphrodisiac, is rich in fish oils and phosphorus.

Ginseng, an Aphrodisiac Herb

Ginseng is used throughout the Orient as a general tonic and panacea reputed to slow the aging process. A Chinese herbalist, Li Chung Yun, drank a daily tea made of ginseng and another Chinese herb (Fo-Ti-Tieng), ate only those vegetables which grew above the ground, drank only mineral water, and maintained a serene attitude at all times. As documented in records kept by the Chinese government, Li Chung Yun lived to be 256 years old (1677–1933)![10]

Ginseng, used before sex, enhances potency. It also helps rebuild energy following exhausting bedroom encounters. Chinese physicians prescribe ginseng as a tonic for general weakness; Soviet astronauts reportedly take ginseng to improve their endurance in space. A number of physicians now employ ginseng for the hot flashes and other discomforts associated with the change of life in women.[11] In such cases, it is used with vitamin E, which may enhance its effect. Chinese herbalists might disapprove of this use, as ginseng traditionally is only for men; by the Chinese science of Yin and Yang, ginseng is the most Yang, or masculine-acting, herb.

The best ginseng reputedly comes from China or Korea. American-grown ginseng isn't as good as the Chinese or Korean but is superior to Japanese. Russian "Siberian ginseng" isn't actually ginseng but rather *Eleutherococcus senticosus*, a more commonly available shrub with properties similar to those of ginseng.

Though available in roots and capsules (from herb shops), the most consistently reliable way to take ginseng is as a tonic. Two extracts I've used and found effective are the Korean Ginseng Extract (imported by Superior Trading Company, San Francisco 94108) and Chinese Panaxum Ginseng, produced at the Chinese Medical Laboratories, Tientsin, China. The usual method of preparation is to put a dose (proper amounts are described on the bottles) in a glass of hot water as a tea. A subtle stimulant effect should be experienced within twenty minutes. If this effect is not observed, the product is too weak or ersatz. Unlike other stimulants, at the recommended dose ginseng doesn't produce nervousness; in fact, it causes relaxation and a feeling of well-being. I sometimes prescribe it as a very mild tranquilizer. Ginseng is best taken on an empty stomach, and fruits should be avoided for three hours after use.

Avoiding Sexual Toxins

Our modern diet is a nutritional disaster. Our grains are first devitalized by grinding away most of their vitamins and minerals; then they are liberally laced with unbalanced proportions of sugar, salt, and various additives. Eating such a highly refined diet may eventually lead to sexual weakness from malnutrition. "Convenience" foods are for the convenience of the food industry. Packaged food is refined and preserved with additives so that it can be shipped great distances and stored on grocery shelves without spoiling. Some recently tested food additives have been shown to cause cancer in rats. Almost three thousand chemicals are approved for use in our food supply; the average American consumes up to nine pounds yearly of these additives.[12] Preservatives are preserving us; unless you want to be a sexual mummy, avoid them.

Even fresh unprocessed foods are inevitably contaminated with herbicide and insecticide residues. Some breast-fed American babies ingest on average ten times more pesticide in mother's milk than the government's maximum acceptable amount. Despite mounting evidence that some pesticides cause cancer, sterility, and birth defects, their use is still increasing. Pesticide use in California doubled between 1974 and 1977.[13] Honey is less likely than most foods to contain insecticide residues simply because bees can't survive them.

Artificial colors are in everything from colored ice cream to hot dogs—even some potatoes. Certain vitamin supplements contain preservatives and artificial sweeteners. Read labels.

Plastic food packaging migrates into food; so we are literally "plastic people." Because it's cheap, plastic is increasingly used to pipe water, though workers in plastics factories have increased amounts of liver cancer. Early senility from aluminum poisoning because of its widespread contact with food is another potential hazard. Lead, our most common pollutant, can cause impotence in men and interfere with fertility in both sexes.

Cigarette smoking decreases sexual strength and sperm production. Offspring of fathers who smoke heavily are less healthy and have twice the amount of congenital malformations.[14] In women, smoking increases the risk of miscarriage and results in smaller-sized babies. Among the several additives in commercial cigarettes is cadmium, which antagonizes zinc and, in excess, stops sperm formation in the testes.

Alcohol, narcotics, and amphetamines used chronically and in excess all lower sexual desire, though the lowering of inhibitions from the moderate use of alcohol may aid lovemaking.

Estrogen compounds decrease sexual desire in both sexes, while androgens (testosterone) increase libido.

Some common medicines interfere with sexual performance. Antihypertensives (Reserpine, Guanethidine, Methyl Dopa) hamper sympathetic response and block ejaculation in men. Certain tranquilizers (Mellaril, Haldol) can retard ejaculation and for that reason have been suggested as a treatment for premature ejaculation. Anticholinergics used to treat glaucoma can obstruct erection.

Caffeine addiction creates a thiamine (vitamin B_1) deficiency, leading to depression and associated loss of sexual interest. Depression and anxiety are perhaps the main sexual "toxins." Along with thiamine, the B vitamins niacin and pyridoxine (B_6) as well as the minerals magnesium and zinc often help hold the "black dog" at bay.

Histamine and Sexual Function

Histamine is a biochemical amine, made by removing the acid group from the amino acid histadine. The intestinal bacteria can split off carbon dioxide (CO_2) from histidine, present in protein foods, and form histamine. A highly active amine,[15] histamine is found in all organic matter, including the body's soft tissues, notably in the brain. In the body, histamine induces the flushing of the allergic reaction and the watery eyes and stuffy nose of the common cold.

Dr. Carl Pfeiffer reports, in a study of twenty-eight males, that their speed of ejaculation was correlated with their blood histamine; the higher the histamine, the quicker the ejaculation.[16] Men too low in histamine cannot attain ejaculation, though erection is no problem. Cells containing histamine are concentrated in the head (glans) of the penis. Similarly, a woman low in histamine may be unable to achieve orgasm and considered frigid. Conversely, men who ejaculate prematurely and women capable of repeated or sustained orgasm may have elevated blood histamine.

The B vitamins folic acid and niacin, because they raise blood histamine, may help men and women low in histamine to reach orgasm. High-histamine men with premature ejaculation are helped by calcium and the amino acid methionine, both of which lower blood histamine.

A Diet for Optimal Sexual Health

Folklore suggests that meat or fish stimulates passion; fish and meat dishes are part of the ancient Tantric sexual ritual. Meat and fish provide complete protein, vital for optimal sexual aggressiveness. It's a matter of Yin and Yang.

Early Chinese philosophers divided all the Universe into two classes, Yin and Yang. The terms first appear in the appendix "Hsi-tz'u" to the *I Ching*, considered to be about 5000 years old. Yang is the virile and Yin the docile principle. Yang is active, masculine, hot, of the Earth. Yin is passive, feminine, cold, of the Heavens.

Our foods fall into one or the other class, with meats and vegetables being predominantly Yang, while sugars, starches, and fruits are mainly Yin. Sex is an active virile Yang act which demands the protein and minerals in meats and vegetables. A diet of fruits and sugar may leave you "spaced out," ethereal, and sensitive, but not sexual. Of course we need both, and eating only Yin or Yang foods throws the body out of balance. As an experiment I once ate an exclusively fruit diet. It made me feel very high, light, and spiritual. I had little interest in sex and became acutely sensitive to the noise and pollution of the city. I stopped after eight days because I was breaking out with acne and having difficulty handling the stress of work.

We should avoid processed and refined foods. Whole unrefined foods provide the vitamins and minerals necessary to metabolize the energy portion of food. Highly refined foods must borrow their missing minerals and vitamins from the body's stores. When these stores become exhausted, the person existing on refined foods becomes exhausted too.

Processing food not only removes nutrients but also the bulk needed to traverse the intestinal tract efficiently. A bulky natural food diet completes its intestinal passage in one-fifth the time of a refined diet. Speedier intestinal transit may explain why heart disease, appendicitis, hemorrhoids, varicose veins, cancer of the colon, and obesity are rare or unknown among African natives living on primitive diets; and also why these ailments are increasingly common in "civilized" nations as we consume more and more processed devitalized food.[17]

A natural foods diet, adequate in protein, vitamins, and minerals, is not only good for sexual vigor but for general health as well. We see that the B vitamins, vitamins C, E, and A, and the essential fatty acids are all required by the sex glands and their hormones. The minerals which seem most important to our sex life are zinc, magnesium, manganese, selenium, and sulfur.

Conclusion

Just as no two of us have the same fingerprints, no two have the same biochemistry. Only by individual biochemical analysis can we determine our unique optimal nutritional need. Yet, we are all enough alike that I can offer some general advice:

(1) Whenever possible, *eat fresh unprocessed food.* Avoid empty calories.

(2) *Breathe deeply of clean air.* Many people have constricted throats and frozen, caved-in chests, respiratory movements stilled by constant subliminal anxiety. Frequently our nostrils are congested from food, coffee, or tobacco allergy. City dwellers often adopt shallow breathing because the air is so polluted that deep breathing could be dangerous.

Our brain in particular needs oxygen; the brain is only 2% of the body's weight but uses 20% of our oxygen. Healthy cells need ample oxygen; cancer cells don't. Cancer cells thrive in low-oxygen environments. Cancer cells are always present in our body, waiting for a foothold. Keeping yourself well oxygenated may prevent their development.

(3) *Drink a mineral-rich (hard) water, free of fluoridation and chlorination.* A recent study indicates a 44% higher incidence of gastrointestinal and urinary tract cancer in populations drinking chlorinated water than in matched groups using non-chlorinated water.

Water fills the stomach, quieting the appetite. It flushes out body poisons and softens the stool, aiding elimination. Many drugs, especially caffeine and alcohol, dehydrate the body. A high protein diet demands water to wash out its nitrogenous waste products.

(4) *Get regular exercise*—jogging, walking, bicycling, sports, dancing, swimming, etc. It helps you sleep, eat, digest

food, and eliminate wastes. Exercise stimulates the circulation, improving the supply of nutrients to the body and aids in removing wastes.

Use common sense; build up your exercise gradually. Don't exercise if you are sick, fasting, or right after eating. Walking is the safest exercise for beginners; if done briskly for extended periods, it is quite effective in exercising the whole body.

Personally, I find exercise for its own sake rather boring. I prefer physical work (gardening, heavy-duty housework, chopping wood, etc.) as a way of getting exercise and also doing something interesting and productive. Spend an hour jogging and you've obtained an hour of exercise. But spend an hour with a shovel turning over the vegetable garden, and you've also gotten your exercise plus accomplished productive work.

(5) *Addiction means malnutrition.* The most common addictions are sugar, salt, coffee, tobacco, and alcohol. Addictions cause four nutritional problems. First, addicting substances are ingested in place of more nutritious foods; or, like cocaine and heroin, they destroy the appetite. Second, some addictions create specific nutritional deficiencies. Caffeine addiction, for example, creates a vitamin B_1 deficiency, cigarettes a vitamin C shortage, etc. Third, toxins in addictive substances place extra nutritional demands. Finally, addictive substances often interfere with intestinal absorption.

(6) *Vitamin supplements provide nutritional insurance.* Here is a daily supplement suitable for most healthy adults:

Vitamin C: 1 g daily with 50 mg of bioflavinoids

B-complex Vitamins:	B_1 (Thiamine)	10 mg
	B_2 (Riboflavin)	10 mg
	B_6 (Pyridoxine)	10 mg
	Niacin	100 mg
	Pantothenic acid	100 mg
	Folic acid	0.5 micrograms
	B_{12} (Cobalamin)	100 micrograms
	Inositol	1 g
	Choline	1 g

Vitamin E (mixed tocopherols): 100 IU for every twenty years of age.

(7) *Stress burns nutrients; remain tranquil.* When stress is unavoidable, supplement generously with vitamin C and the B-complex.

If you have symptoms described in this book, *don't* attempt self-treatment. Seek out a physician experienced in the use of nutrients; they are a small but increasing number. Perhaps your physician is knowledgeable about nutrition and vitamin therapy. If not, you might make him a present of this book.

Nutrition and vitamin therapy is a new science. Some of its practitioners are outstanding, some mediocre, and a few disappointing. I have a dream that someday all physicians will turn first to nutrients when treating and preventing disease. That will require a small revolution in medicine. But Hippocrates, the father of medicine, said: *"Let thy food be thy medicine and thy medicine be thy food."*

Physicians need to recognize that a sick patient is often a hungry and/or a chemically poisoned patient. Thousands, victims of ignorance, languish in mental hospitals with undiagnosed chemical pollution or malnutrition. May the modern psychiatrist return to the full practice of medicine which his patients so badly need. *Every disease has a real cause. No disease is all in your mind.*

The chemical hazards of our environment and the absence of nourishment in our diet are alarming. But only if we recognize the *real* dangers and work to correct our spoiled Eden can we hope to survive.

It is not too late. We can clean up the air, the water, and our food chain. It's a simple choice of life or death. Choose life.

References

Chapter Two

1. Kanehiro Takaki, "Health of the Imperial Japanese Navy," *Lancet* 2 (1887): 86, 189, 233.
2. Prevost and Maffoni, *Acad. Sci. Med.* 3 (Turin, 1846): 453.
3. Casimir Funk, "On the Chemical Nature of the Substance Which Cures Polyneuritis in Birds Induced by a Diet of Polished Rice," *Journal of Physiology* 43 (1911): 395–400.
4. William Kaufman, *The Common Form of Joint Dysfunction: Its Incidence and Treatment* (Brattleboro, Vt.: E. L. Hildreth and Co., 1949).
5. F.R. Klenner, "The Treatment of Poliomyelitis and Other Viral Diseases with Vitamin C," *Southern Medicine and Surgery* 111 (1949): 209–214.
6. John F.J. Cade, "Lithium Salts in the Treatment of Psychotic Excitement," *Medical Journal of Australia* 36 (1949): 349.
7. H. Osmond and A. Hoffer, "Massive Niacin Treatment in Schizophrenia," *Lancet* 1 (10 February 1962): 316–319.
8. Michael Lesser, *Depression and Blood Cortisol* (New York, N.Y.: Cornell University Medical College, December 1963). Unpublished.
9. Michael Lesser, *A Social Systems Approach to the Treatment of Narcotics Addicts* (Washington, D.C.: Clinical Society of U. S. Public Health Service, 1969).
10. Ida P. Rolf, *Rolfing* (New York: Harper & Row, 1977).

11. *Diet Related to Killer Diseases, V*, Hearing before the U.S. Senate Select Committee on Nutrition and Human Needs, Mental Health and Mental Development, June 22, 1977 (Washington, D.C.: U. S. Government Printing Office, 1977).

Chapter Three

Thiamine
1. R. Williams, H.L. Mason, B.F. Smith, and R.M. Wilder, "Induced Thiamine (B₁) Deficiency and the Thiamine Requirement of Man," *Archives of Internal Medicine* 69, no. 5 (May 1942): 721–738.

Niacin
2. "Maise Mystery," *Medical Newsmagazine* 22, no. 4 (April 1968): 147–151.
3. Health and Nutrition Examination Survey (HANES), U.S. Department of Health, Education and Welfare, 1971–1972.

Pyridoxine
4. C.C. Pfeiffer et al., "Treatment of Pyroluric Schizophrenia (Malvaria) with Large Doses of Pyridoxine and a Dietary Supplement of Zinc," *The Journal of Orthomolecular Psychiatry* 3, no. 4 (1974): 292–300.
5. B. Rimland, E. Callaway, and P. Dreyfus, "The Effect of High Doses of Vitamin B₆ on Autistic Children: A Double-Blind Crossover Study," *American Journal of Psychiatry* 135, no. 4 (April 1978): 472–475.
6. E.L. Prien and S.F. Gershoff, "Magnesium Oxide-Pyridoxine Therapy for Recurrent Calcium Oxalate Calculi," *Journal of Urology* 112, no. 4 (October 1974): 509–12.
7. P.W. Adams et al., "Effect of Pyridoxine Hydrochloride (Vitamin B₆) Upon Depression Associated with Oral Contraception," *Lancet* 1 (28 April 1973): 899–904.
8. John Ellis, *Vitamin B₆, The Doctor's Report* (New York: Harper & Row, 1973).
9. U. Ottersdorf et al., "Interactions of Non-Nutrients with Nutrients," *World Review of Nutrition and Dietetics* 26 (Basel: Karger, 1977): 4–134.

Pantothenic Acid

10. Gordon, "Pantothenic Acid in Human Nutrition," *Symposium on Biological Action Vitamins* (Chicago: University of Chicago, 1942): 136–143.
11. Emmanual Cheraskin and W.M. Ringsdorf, "Bruxism: A Nutritional Problem?" *Dental Survey* (December 1970): 38, 40.
12. *Proceedings of the Society of Biology* 86 (1954).
13. R.J. Williams, *Nutrition Against Disease* (New York: Pitman Publishing, 1971).

Cobalamin

14. F.R. Ellis and S. Nasser, "A Pilot Study of B_{12} in the Treatment of Tiredness," *British Journal of Nutrition* 30 (1973): 277–283.
15. H. Wieck, W. Pribilla, and B. Heerklotz, "Psychoses as a Manifestation of B_{12} Deficiency," *Deutsche Medizinische Wochenschrift* 94 (1969): 1973.
16. C.C. Pfeiffer, *Mental and Elemental Nutrients* (New Canaan, Conn.: Keats Publishing, 1975).

Folic Acid

17. J. Rose, "Folic Acid as a Cause of Angular Cheilosis," *Lancet* 2 (1971): 453.
18. *New England Journal of Medicine* (16 October 1975).
19. *Lancet* (9 August 1975).
20. E. Reynolds, J. Preece, and A. Johnson, "Folate Metabolism in Epileptic and Psychiatric Patients," *Journal of Neurology, Neurosurgery and Psychiatry* 34 (1971): 726.

Choline

21. Kenneth L. Davis, Leo E. Hollister, Jack D. Barchas, and Philip A. Berger, "Choline in Tardive Dyskinesia and Huntington's Disease," *Life Sciences* 19 (1976): 1507–1516.
22. *Journal of Vitaminology* 3 (1957): 106.

Botin

23. V.P. Sydenstricker et al., "Observations on 'Egg White Injury in Man and Its Cure with Biotin Concentrate,' " *Science* 95 (1942): 176–177; *Journal of The American Medical Association* 118 (1942): 1199–1200.

Pangamic Acid
24. E.D. Michlin, ed., *Vitamin B₁₅ Properties, Functions and Use* (Moscow: Science Publishing House, 1965). Reprinted by Cancer Book House, Los Angeles.

Chapter Four

1. Irwin Stone, *The Healing Factor, "Vitamin C" Against Disease* (New York: Grossett & Dunlap, 1972).
2. H. Vanderkamp, "A Biochemical Abnormality in Schizophrenia Involving Ascorbic Acid," *International Journal of Neurochemistry and Psychiatry* 2 (1966): 204–206.
3. A.E. Libby and Irwin Stone, "The Hypoascorbemia-Kwashiorkor Approach to Drug Addiction Therapy: A Pilot Study," *Journal of Orthomolecular Psychiatry* 6, no. 4 (1977).
4. Joseph Borkin, *The Crime and Punishment of I.G. Farben* (New York: Macmillan Publishing Co., 1978).
5. A.L. Kubala and M.M. Katz, "Nutritional Factors in Psychological Test Behavior," *Journal of Genetic Psychology* 96 (1960): 343–352.
6. Linus Pauling, "Orthomolecular Medicine," *Nutrition Today,* March–April 1978.
7. F.R. Klenner (with F.H. Bartz), *The Key to Good Health: Vitamin C* (Chicago, Ill.: Graphic Arts Research Foundation, 1969).
8. J. Greenwood, "Optimum Vitamin C Intake as a Factor in the Preservation of Disc Integrity," *Medical Annals of the District of Columbia* 33 (1965): 274–276.
9. Linus Pauling, *Vitamin C, the Common Cold, and the Flu* (San Francisco: W.H. Freeman & Co., 1976).
10. Ewan Cameron and Linus Pauling, *Proceedings National Academy of Science* 73, no. 10 (October 1976): 3685–3689.
11. Robert Cathcart, *Proceedings Orthomolecular Medical Society,* 2nd Annual Meeting, San Francisco, February 1977 (Pasadena, Calif.: Instatape).
12. Thomas F. Dowd, *Science News Letter* 17 (January 1959).
13. Edme Regnier, "The Administration of Large Doses of Ascorbic Acid in the Prevention and Treatment of the

Common Cold, Parts I and II," *Review of Allergy* 22 (1968): 835–846, 948–956.

Chapter Five

Vitamin A

1. Adelle Davis, *Let's Eat Right to Keep Fit* (New York: Harcourt, Brace & World, 1954), p. 51.
2. H.R. Cama, N.C. Pillai, P.R. Sundareson, and C. Venkateshan, "The Effect of Thyroid Activity on the Conversion of Carotene and Retinene to Vitamin A and on Serum Proteins," *Journal of Nutrition* 63 (1957): 571.
3. M.S. Robboy et al., "The Hypercarotenemia of Anorexia Nervosa: A Comparison of Vitamin A and Carotene Levels in Various Forms of Menstrual Dysfunction and Cachexia," *American Journal of Clinical Nutrition* 27 (1974): 362–367.
4. W.J. Kinley and R.F. Krause, "Influence of Vitamin A on Cholesterol Blood Units," *Proceedings of the Society for Experimental Biology and Medicine* 102 (1959): 353.
5. Michael Sporn, National Cancer Institute Research Center Workshop, February, 1978, Bethesda, Maryland, and in *American Medical News* 235 (5 April 1976): 1409.

Vitamin D

6. J.Y. Moon, "A Macrobiotic Explanation of Pathological Calcification," *G.D.M.F.*, San Francisco, 1974.
7. H. Selye, *Calciphylaxsis* (Chicago: University of Chicago Press, 1962).
8. W.W. Meyer, "Calcifications of the Carotid Siphon—a Common Finding in Infancy and Childhood," *Archives of Disease in Childhood* 47 (June 1972): 355–363.
9. C. Reich, "Allergy and Diseases of the Central Nervous System," *Journal of Orthomolecular Psychiatry* 4, no. 4 (1975): 269–273.

Vitamin E

10. N.R. Kavinoky, "Vitamin E and Control of Climacteric Symptoms," *Annals of Western Medicine and Surgery* 4 (1950): 27–32.

11. L. Packer and J.R. Smith, *Medical World News*, 25 October 1974.

12. *Nutrition Today* (January 1972).

13. W.E. Shute, "Chapter 69: The Vitamin E Story," in *The Complete Book of Vitamins*, ed. C. Gerras (Emmaus, Pa.: Rodale Press, 1977).

Chapter Six

1. F.P. Antia, *Clinical Dietetics and Nutrition* (New York: Oxford University Press, 1966).

2. J.I. Rodale, "Chapter 7," in *The Complete Book of Minerals* (Emmaus, Pa.: Rodale Books, 1977).

3. F. Flack, *British Journal of Psychiatry* 116 (1970): 437–438.

4. Susanna Denes, "Disturbances of Calcium and Phosphorus Metabolism in Premature Old Age," *Journal of the American Geriatrics Society* 15 (October 1967): 941–947.

5. Alice Bernheim, "A Calcium Regimen in Allergy," *Annals of Allergy* 22 (September 1964): 449–459.

6. T.J. Hahn et al., *Archives of Gynecology*, 213 (1972): 176–186.

7. J. Lemann et al., "Evidence That Glucose Ingestion Inhibits Net Renal Tubular Reabsorption of Calcium and Magnesium in Man," *Journal of Laboratory and Clinical Medicine* 75, no. 4 (1970): 578–585.

8. J. Lemann, et al., *Journal Dairy Science* 26, no. 10 (1943): 951–958.

9. A.D. Newcomer and D.B. McGill, "Disaccharidase Activity in the Small Intestine: Prevalence of Lactase Deficiency in 100 Healthy Subjects," *Gastroenterology* 53 (1967): 881–889.

10. D. Frizel et al., *British Journal of Psychiatry* 115 (529), pp. 1375–1377.

11. D. Frizel et al., *American Journal of Medical Sciences* 237 (1959): 413–417.

12. D. Frizel et al., *Soviet Medicine* 34, no. 5 (1971): 140–142.

13. R.H. Seller et al., "Magnesium Metabolism in Hypertension," *Journal of the American Medical Association* 191, no. 3 (1965): 654–656.

14. Mildred Seelig, "The Requirement of Magnesium by the Normal Adult," *American Journal of Clinical Nutrition* 14 (June 1964): 242–290.

15. D. Hingerty, "The Role of Magnesium in Adrenal Insufficiency," *Biochemical Journal* 66 (July 1957): 429–431.

16. Paul J. Schecter, David Horowitz, and Robert I. Henkin, "Sodium Chloride Preference in Essential Hypertension," *Journal of the American Medical Association* 225 (10 September 1973): 1311–1315.

17. G. Spergel et al., *Metabolism, Clinical and Experimental* 16, no. 17 (1967): 581–585.

18. R. Ishigami et al., *Proceedings of Third Asia and Oceania Congress of Endocrinology*, Jan. 2–6, 1967.

19. A.J. Swallow, "The Action of α-Radiation on Aqueous Solutions of Cysteine," *Journal of The Chemical Society* 243 (London, 1952): 1334.

20. R.C. Jain, "Effect of Garlic on Serum Lipids, Coagulability, and Fibrinolytic Activity of Blood," *American Journal of Clinical Nutrition* 30 (September 1977): 1380–1381.

Chapter Seven

1. S.A.K. Wilson, "Progressive Lenticular Degeneration: A Familial Nervous Disease Associated with Cirrhosis of The Liver," *Brain* 34 (1911–12): 295–509.

2. Carl C. Pfeiffer, M.D., and Venelin Iliev, "A Study of Zinc Deficiency and Copper Excess in the Schizophrenias," *International Review of Neurobiology*, Supplement 1 (London, 1972).

3. William R. Beisel and Robert S. Pekarek, "Acute Stress and Trace Element Metabolism," *International Review of Neurobiology*, Supplement 1 (London, 1972): 53–82.

4. Ananda Prasad, *Zinc Metabolism* (Springfield Ill.: Charles C. Thomas, 1966).

5. G. Michaelsson, "Effects of Oral Zinc and Vitamin A in Acne," *Archives for Dermatology* 113 (January 1977): 31.

6. P.J. Schechter and R.I. Henkin et al., "Idiopathic Hypo-

geusia: A Description of the Syndrome and A Single-Blind Study with Zinc Sulfate," *International Review of Neurobiology,* Supplement 1 (London, 1972): 125–140.

7. J.V. Murphy, "Intoxication Following Ingestion of Elemental Zinc," *Journal of the American Medical Association* 212, no. 12 (1970): 2119.

8. M.L. Taylor et al. *Journal of the American Medical Association* 187, no. 5 (1964): 323–327.

9. M.L. Taylor et al., *Journal of Pediatrics* 86, no. 4 (1975): 542–547.

10. M.L. Taylor et al., *Haematologia* 5, no. 4 (1971): 369–375.

11. L.G. Kosenko, "Soderzhanie Nekotorykh Mikroélementov v Krovi Bol'nykh Sakharnym Diabetom," *Klinische Medizine* 42 (1964): 113–116.

12. Ruth Adams and Frank Murray, *Minerals: Kill or Cure?* (New York: Larchmont Books, 1974).

13. Richard Kunin, "Manganese and Niacin in the Treatment of Drug-Induced Dyskinesias," *Journal of Orthomolecular Psychiatry* 5, no. 1 (1976): 4–27.

14. Henry A. Schroeder, *The Trace Elements and Man* (Old Greenwich, Conn.: The Devin-Adair Company, 1973).

15. Henry A. Schroeder, *Pollution, Profits and Progress* (Brattleboro, Vt.: The Stephen Greene Press, 1971).

16. Carl C. Pfeiffer, *Zinc and Other Micronutrients* (New Canaan, Conn.: Keats Publishing, 1978).

17. E.M. Trautner et al., "The Excretion and Retention of Ingested Lithium and Its Effect on the Ionic Balance of Man," *Medical Journal of Australia* 42 (1955): 280.

18. Trevor R.P. Price and Paul J. Beisswenger, "Lithium and Diabetes Insipidus," *Annals of Internal Medicine* 88, no. 4 (April 1978): 576–577.

19. Gosta Bucht and Anders Wahlin, "Impairment of Renal Concentrating Capacity by Lithium," *Lancet* 1, no. 8067 (8 April 1976): 778–779.

20. H.L. Meltzer et al., "Rubidium: A Potential Modifier of Affect and Behavior," *Nature* 223 (1969): 321–322.

21. Ronald R. Fieve, Paper given at World Congress of Biological Psychiatry, August 31–September 8, 1978, Barcelona, Spain.

Chapter Eight

1. Henry A. Schroeder, *The Trace Elements and Man* (Old Greenwich, Conn.: The Devin-Adair Company, 1973).

2. *Minerals Yearbook,* Vol. 1, U.S. Department of the Interior, prepared by the staff of the Bureau of Mines (Washington, D.C.; U. S. Government Printing Office, 1970).

3. Anthony Tucker, *The Toxic Metals* (London: Earth Island Limited, 1972).

4. S.H. Lamm and J.F. Rosen, "Lead Contamination in Milks Fed to Infants: 1972–1973," *Pediatrics* 53 (1974): 137.

5. *Lead: Airborne Lead in Perspective* (Washington, D.C.: National Research Council–National Academy of Sciences, 1972).

6. P.S.I. Berry and D.B. Mossman, "Lead Concentration in Human Tissue," *British Journal of Industrial Medicine* 27 (1970): 339.

7. Henry A. Schroeder and I.H. Tipton, "The Human Body Burden of Lead," *Archives of Environmental Health* 17 (1968): 965–978.

8. Oliver David et al., "Lead and Hyperactivity," *Lancet* 2 (1972): 900–903.

9. D. Bryce-Smith and H.A. Waldrin, "Lead, Behavior and Criminality," *The Ecologist* 4, no. 10, December 1974.

10. D. Bryce-Smith and H.A. Waldrin, "Lead Pollution—A Growing Hazard to Public Health," *Chemistry in Britain* 7 (February 1971): 254–256.

11. W.J. Niklowitz and D.W. Yeager, "Interference of Pb with Essential Brain Tissue Cu, Fe and Zn as Main Determinant in Experimental Tetraethyllead Encephalopathy," *Life Science* 13 (1973): 897–905.

12. L. Kocsar, L. Kedztyus et al., *Acta Physiologica Academiae Scientiarum Hungaricae* 5 (1954): 531, 537, 543.

13. M.N. Valloton, M. Guilleman, and M. Lob, "Plombémie et Activité de la Déhydratase de l'Acide-Aminolévulinique dans une Population Lausannoise," *Schweizerisches Medezinische Wochenschrift* 103 (1973): 547–550.

14. K.M. Six and R.A. Goyer, "Experimental Enhancement of Lead Toxicity by Low Dietary Calcium," *Journal of Laboratory and Clinical Medicine* 76 (1970): 933.

15. R. Kunin, "Lead Toxicity, A Clinical Challenge," Congress of Orthomolecular Psychiatry and Medicine, San Diego, September, 1978.

16. *Minamata Disease* (Japan: Kumamoto University, 1968).

17. J.I. Rodale, *The Complete Book of Minerals for Health* (Emmaus, Pa.: Rodale Books, 1977).

18. H. Petering and L. Tepper, "Pharmacology and Tox. of Heavy Metals: Mercury," *Pharm. Ther. A.* 1 (1976): 131–151.

19. Elizabeth L. Rees, "Report on Trace Metals in Hair," *Diet Related To Killer Diseases V* (Washington, D.C.: U. S. Government Printing Office, 1977), p. 245.

20. "Arsenic-Lead Synergism," translated in *Journal of Hygiene and Sanitation* 34 (Moscow: Ministry of Health, 1969): 123.

21. L. Kopeloff, S. Barrera, and N. Kopeloff, "Recurrent Convulsive Seizures in Animals Produced by Immunologic and Chemical Means," *American Journal of Psychiatry* 98 (1942): 881–902.

22. I. Klatzo, H. Wisniewski, and J. Streicher, "Experimental Production of Neurofibrillary Degeneration," *Journal of Neuropathology and Experimental Neurology* 24 (1965): 187–199.

23. D.R. Crapper, S.S. Krishman, and A.J. Dalton, "Brain Aluminum Distribution and Experimental Distribution and Experimental Neuro-fibrillary Degeneration," *Science* (May 1973): 180.

24. C.C. Pfeiffer, *Zinc and Other Micronutrients* (New Canaan: Conn.: Keats Publishing Company, 1978).

25. Lawrence C. Kolb, *Noyes' Modern Clinical Psychiatry* (Philadelphia: W.B. Saunders, 1968).

26. David C. Hilderbrand and Darl H. White, "Trace Element Analysis in Hair: An Evaluation," *Clinical Chemistry* 20 (1974): 148–151.

Chapter Nine

1. G.M. Beard, "Nutrition or Nervous Exhaustion," *Boston Medical and Surgical Journal* 57 (1869): 217.

2. G.M. Beard, *A Practical Treatise on Nervous Exhaustion* (New York: William Wood, 1880).

3. S. Freud, "Sexuality in the Etiology of the Neuroses" (1898), in *Collection of Papers*, Vol. I (London: Hogarth, 1950), p. 240.

4. S. Freud, "The Justification for Detachment from Neurasthenia a Particular Syndrome: The Anxiety Neurosis," in *Collection of Papers*, Vol. 1 (London: Hogarth, 1950), pp. 75, 106.

5. S. Harris, "Hyperinsulinism and Dysinsulinism," *Journal of the American Medical Association* 83 (1924): 289–733.

6. F. Alexander and S.A. Portis, "A Psychosomatic Study of Hypoglycemic Fatigue," *Psychosomatic Medicine* 6 (1944): 191–205.

7. G. Heninger and P. Mueller, "Carbohydrate Metabolism in Mania," *Archives of General Psychiatry* 23 (1970): 330–339.

8. R. Peterson and R. Stillman, eds., *Cocaine, 1977*, Department of Health, Education and Welfare, Public Health Service NIDA Reseach Monograph #13, Rockville Maryland, 1977.

9. S. Bernfeld, "Freud's Studies on Cocaine," in *Cocaine Papers: Sigmund Freud*, ed. R. Byck (New York: Stonehill Publishing Co., 1974).

10. D. Musto, *The American Disease—Origins of Narcotic Control* (New Haven: Yale University Press, 1973).

11. Lawrence Dickey, ed., *Clinical Ecology* (Springfield, Ill.: Charles C. Thomas, 1976).

12. E.W. Abrahamson and A.W. Pezet, *Body, Mind, and Sugar* (New York: Holt, Rinehart and Winston, 1951).

Chapter Ten

1. Arthur F. Coca, *The Pulse Test; Easy Allergy Detection* (New York: Arco Publishing Co., 1977).

2. Hans Selye, *The Stress of Life* (New York: McGraw-Hill Book Company, 1956).

3. Adelle Davis, *Let's Get Well* (New York: Harcourt Brace Jovanovich, 1965).

Chapter Eleven

1. Paavo O. Airola, *Sex and Nutrition* (New York: Award Books, 1970).
2. Hans Selye, *The Stress of Life* (New York: McGraw-Hill Book Company, 1956).
3. G.V. Mann et al., "Cardiovascular Disease in the Masai," *Journal of Atherosclerosis Research* 4 (1964): 289.
4. Robert C. Kolodny et al., "Depression of Plasma Testosterone Levels after Chronic Intensive Marihuana Use," *The New England Journal of Medicine* 290, no. 16 (18 April 1974): 872–874.
5. J. Janick et al., "Seminal Fluid and Spermatozoon Motility," *Fertility and Sterility* 22, no. 9 (1971): 573–589.
6. Barbara and Gideon Seaman, "Chapter Six" in *Women and the Crisis in Sex Hormones* (New York: Rawson Associates, 1977).
7. Barbara and Gideon Seaman, "Chapter Eight" in *Women and the Crisis in Sex Hormones* (New York: Rawson Associates, 1977).
8. Daphne A. Roe, "How the Pill Affects a Woman's Nutritional Status," *Medical Opinion* (September 1976): 58–61.
9. John Lindenbaum et al., "Oral Contraceptive Hormones, Folate Metabolism, and the Cervical Epithelium," *American Journal of Clinical Nutrition* 28 (1975): 346–352.
10. Sarah Harriman, *The Book of Ginseng* (New York: Pyramid Books, 1973).
11. Barbara and Gideon Seaman, "Chapter 31" in *Women and the Crisis in Sex Hormones* (New York: Rawson Associates, 1977).
12. Victor F. Zonana, "More Foods Today Are 'Fresh' from Factories and Quick to Prepare," *The Wall Street Journal*, 21 June 1977.
13. Marcy Damovsky, "Who Killed George Neary's Cows?" *Berkeley Barb*, 29 March 1979.
14. Alton Ochsner, "Adverse Effect of Smoking on Sexuality," *Medical Aspects of Human Sexuality* (March 1976): 15.
15. Gale, *Advances in Enzymology* 6 (1946): 1.

16. Carl C. Pfeiffer, *Mental and Elemental Nutrients* (New Canaan, Conn.: Keats Publishing, 1975).
17. S. Wapnick et al., "Can Diet Be Responsible for the Initial Lesion in Diabetes?" *Lancet* 2 (12 August 1972): 300.

Index

Aangamik 15 (vitamin supplement), 65
Abrahamson, E. W., 177
Academy of Orthomolecular Psychiatry, 31, 32
acanthosis nigricans, 49
acne, 54, 90, 129, 167, 200
acne rosacea, 40
ACTH, 194
adrenal glands and hormones, 22, 56, 78, 91, 114, 117, 118, 174, 175, 176–77, 188–89, 190, 194, 195–96
aging, 58, 60, 64, 65, 72, 79, 91, 99–100, 110, 133, 194
   See also Senility
air pollution, 9, 72, 76, 77, 95, 96, 99, 101, 147, 148, 151, 156, 211
alcohol abuse, xiii, 4, 12, 13, 40, 130, 131, 149, 151, 182, 186, 187, 189, 196, 201, 208, 211, 212
   and hypoglycemia, 171, 173, 175
   vitamin depletion in, 39, 61, 112, 113
   vitamin therapy for, 49, 65, 74, 112
alcoholic polyneuritis, 39
alcoholic psychosis, 56
Alexander, Franz, 168–70
alienation, 124
allergies, 5, 32, 56, 110, 130

   See also Food addictions and allergies
aluminum contamination, 123, 150, 153–54, 159, 208
   case history, 153–54
   and mind, 155
   sources of, 153, 155–56
   of water, 155
Alvarez, Walter, 179–80, 181
Alzheimer's disease, 155
American Heart Journal, 197
American Psychiatric Association, 33
   Task Force Report #7, 32
American Schizophrenia Association, 31
Ames Medical Laboratory, 77
amphetamines, 189, 208
anemia, 60, 78, 79, 101, 131, 132, 133
   iron-resistant, 52, 53, 54
   pernicious, 57, 58
anger, 12, 124
anorexia nervosa, 92, 183–84
antibiotics, 21, 79, 90–91, 105, 189
antihistamines, 49, 189
anxiety, 2–4, 73, 90, 97, 109, 112, 115, 166, 209
aphrodisiacs, 205–06
   See also specific foods
Arfvedson, J. A., 138
armoring, 31, 175
arsenic, 72, 123, 137, 150, 159, 202

ABOUT THE AUTHOR

MICHAEL LESSER, M.D., a leading practitioner of nutritional medicine, is a psychiatrist trained at Cornell Medical School and the Albert Einstein Medical School in New York. He currently practices in Berkeley, California.